PRAISE FOR SHARRY EDWARDS AND HUMAN BIOACOUSTICS

Sharry Edwards is a true pioneer in the field of Sound Healing. The sound frequency-based diagnostic and therapeutic protocols she has developed as the founder of Human BioAcoustics has the potential to completely revolutionize medicine as we know it, and for the better! I encourage you to read *Breaking the Sound Barrier of Disease* to learn how you can use Sharry›s methods to quickly, noninvasively, and effectively improve your health and the health of your loved ones.

~ **Michael Karlfeldt, ND, PhD, founder of The Karlfeldt Center and bestselling author of *A Better Way To Treat Cancer***

Long before the term "sound healing" was coined, Sharry Edwards heard sounds from people that you and I cannot hear. These tones are not a product of a fanciful imagination, but have been confirmed by scientists. What does she hear that we don't? She hears your body sending signals from your ears to another part of your body. These signals are sounds your body needs to heal.

Everything in our body is energy and therefore has its own frequency. Sharry focused on it. Certain sounds were a repeatable response to a disease. What a discovery! Furthermore, she could vocalize sounds and watch the body heal. Her dogged perseverance led her to this and many more groundbreaking discoveries, which premier medical facilities are now scrambling to replicate.

With compassion for others, Sharry shares her gifts with the world, not just by devising healing sounds for you, but also providing tools to access the communication of your subtle body signals. She developed software and methods to detect the tonal signals that allow your body to heal itself. She gave individuals, like you and me, the power to learn about their bodies, what they genuinely need, and mechanisms to deliver the necessary tones to their bodies.

Typically, today, we identify what the body needs through symptoms, and we verify our guesses with testing. That is time-consuming and expensive; maybe we are testing the wrong thing, or perhaps the medical field doesn't have a cure. Sound, however, can be measured, revealing precisely what is "out of tune" in your body—getting rid of the guesswork.

From personal empowerment to hope for incurable problems and affordable solutions, Sharry offers it all.

~ Jill Mattson, Musician, Composer, Author, and Intuitive

There is an unseen extension of the physical world which, as 'The Music of the Spheres', bring healing properties from subtle planetary regions into the material world. This directly confirms Sharry Edwards research, which prompted me to identify her as a 'Scientist of the Grail.' Her discoveries have been further corroborated by scientists with the aid of the latest high-speed computers. Her work could provide a necessary paradigm for a unifying field theory of subtle energy medicine.

~ Sylvia Franke, author of *The Tree of Life and the Holy Grail*

Prevention and early detection of disease are becoming the patient-preferred, new paradigm for healthcare. As such, voice analysis technology that can both detect and monitor the progression of health issues gives healthcare providers the ability to remotely discern the subtle changes in speech, pitch, rate and breath patterns. This data can pinpoint the potential and the progression of a patient's dis-ease. Most importantly, it is done without the use of toxic chemicals or tests and procedures that are both costly and come with their own risk profiles.

From a holistic perspective, the voice print analysis and other Human BioAcoustic technology developed by Sharry Edwards could revolutionize healthcare methods of diagnosis, risk assessment and the management of symptoms and clinical outcomes. Instead of isolating the symptoms of a particular body system's malfunction, voice analysis uses biomarkers that incorporate both emotional and psychological factors, to provide an integrated presentation of the patient's overall health status.

Breaking the Sound Barrier of Disease is a must read for those who have eyes to see and ears to hear. It contains valuable information that could permanently alter the landscape of healthcare in the future, by providing both patients and their providers a practical resource to promote health, healing, and holistic well being.

~ **Gwen Olsen, Author** *of Confessions of an Rx Drug Pusher*

Having an idea to create something genuinely new in the world is one thing. Actually doing it and bringing it to fruition as something that helps the world is another. Sharry Edwards is a gifted, uniquely talented woman who has done this for the healing of everyone, bringing together sound, music, chemistry, and physics to create a modality and technology that I have seen create small and big miracles. Her BioAcoustic Math Matrix work is taking us into the future of medicine and offers a new, clear vision of how to help the body use its innate ability to heal using frequency at various octave ranges and in unique wave form patterns to bring sound to matter. Not as magic but as science.

~ **Anita Vanderhaeghe, President, Delphi Consulting**

I was a real skeptic at first—Human BioAcoustics seemed too good to be true. After seeing my son Willie's progress, however, I believe that Sound Health is on the periphery of the greatest discovery ever made concerning treatment of the human body."

~ **William Crum, Governor's appointee to the Ohio State Independent Living Council**

I was involved in a motorcycle accident that destroyed my lower leg. The medical establishment wanted to amputate but I refused. After two years of surgeries and rehab, my leg was still not functional. The doctors told me that my life was never going to be the same. There was no more help they could provide. My future prospects for my love of tennis and physical activity looked bleak.

By a total quirk of fate, I met Sharry Edward's husband at our local grocery. I guess the tennis logo on my shirt and my obvious disability led him to approach me about a protocol for injured muscles. Honestly, I just thought he was a bit off but he invited me to hit practice balls with him on his personal tennis court, so I agreed. I explained that I couldn't move fast or quick but he assured me that he could hit the ball to me and at least I could rally even if I couldn't run.

As the session went on, my pain levels rose to the point that I could not continue. As we were talking afterwards, and unbeknownst to me, Sharry started playing a non-intrusive ambient sound from a machine that sounded like background noise. Within minutes I began to notice that my pain was subsiding. The proof of what her husband had told me about Sharry's unique sound healing talents was right in front of me.

Not having to deal with constant pain and loads of pain medication was a welcoming thought. I agreed to provide a vocal print to Sharry for her research. From the frequencies of my voice, she was able to determine the lower leg muscle sounds that I needed. I played the sounds to reduce the pain but my leg rehabilitated itself and has returned to its normal form and function.

I find the thought of frequency healing to be improbable but I'm proof that it works. I'm now back to playing tennis, even coaching some high level players. Sharry's techniques work. She gave me back my life and I will be forever grateful. So will millions of others if her techniques are ever allowed to become a part of mainstream medicine and everyday life.

~ **Robert Bethel, JD**

BREAKING *the*
SOUND BARRIER
of DISEASE

How the Healing Power of Sound Can Restore Your Health and Transform the Future of Medicine

Sharry Edwards, MEd
Larry Trivieri Jr

Library of Congress Cataloging-in-Publication Data has been applied for.
ISBN: 978-0-9631878-5-7 (hardcover)
ISBN: 978-0-9631878-7-1 (trade paperback)
ISBN: 978-0-9631878-8-8 (ebook)

Book Cover Design and Interior Formatting by 100Covers.

CONTENTS

DEDICATION

To my children, Rickii, Ronna and Jesse, who had to do with a mother for sometimes months at a time while I was on the road, my sincere appreciation and apology.

And to my husband, William, who held me together during the bad times. No amount of thanks could ever repay you for allowing me to live this life of exploration and expansion.

"The doctor of the future is the patient."

~ Dr. Sachin Patel

INTRODUCTION— SHARRY EDWARDS SAVED MY LIFE BY JAMES MARSHALL

I am a spiritual actor, composer, and performer. Such was not always my path. I had always wanted to be a part of the Hollywood scene and by the start of the 1990s, I was finally reaching the peak of my career. I had a role on the television show, Twin Peaks, and was cast in numerous roles in films, including A Few Good Men, starring Tom Cruise, Jack Nicholson, and Demi Moore; Cadence, starring Martin Sheen and Charlie Sheen; Gladiator, starring Cuba Gooding Jr. I thought this was the beginning of a wonderful career when all of a sudden it had to be put on hold.

I thought my life would end after taking the advice of a conventional medical provider, and it almost did. The medicine that was prescribed to me destroyed my large intestine to the point where it had to be removed. After nearly two years of being bed-ridden in a hospital room, I weighed less than 100 pounds and my lack of energy and bad health had ended my acting career.

One fateful night, I was up late searching for an answer. I began to listen to the Coast-to-Coast radio show. George Noory was interviewing a woman about a healing technique that she had been developing using sound frequencies. Her name is Sharry Edwards. Research that was being conducted on Human BioAcoustics, which Sharry developed, was showing that sound could heal people. You simply had to find the right sound frequency and match it to the person.

After listening to Sharry talk about her work, I took a chance and called her research center. After hearing my story, she agreed to help. She used her own computer software to analyze my voice and it created a report on my health status. This report indicated which vitamins and nutrients I needed to help my body heal itself. Then I was told which foods might provide this for me and which foods I should avoid. Along with this I was given sound frequencies that might, theoretically, help to heal me as well.

Sharry gave me a list of individualized frequencies which I recreated using my guitar. Not musical notes, but frequencies that could be tuned. It didn't sound exactly like music, but it was incredibly pleasing to me. I spent long hours with the sounds. I began to feel more and more like my old self. Since then, I've learned that our DNA is basically frequency, and it can be set to music. Was I using music to speak to my DNA in a way that caused my body to heal itself?

I started to gain weight, and my energy returned. I spent hours with the sounds, and I began to feel like my old self.

I became so fascinated at my own progress using sound that my wife, Renee, and I began to study, in depth, ancient techniques of sound healing that were being brought into the modern era by Sharry's novel research. When I learned that all of this stemmed from Sharry's innate ability to hear and duplicate sounds that were unlike normal human abilities, I knew that I wanted to be part of bringing this "other dimensional" talent of hers to the forefront of health and wellness. She was very open to my ideas.

I wanted to work on something significant, something timely, something useful to the public. We chose the threat of the pandemic swine flu. Sharry decoded the genetic make-up of the different strains of swine flu (as she had done for so many other pathogens) and, using extrapolations from her previous research, she came up with the frequency biomarkers for the swine flu. She was also able to mathematically determine the frequency-based antidotes.

When I received the set of frequencies from Sharry's research lab, I was perplexed. These were not notes that one would play together harmonically. I could not see a way that these notes could be combined into a pleasing musical piece. But I believed in the magic of what she had done for me. I had to give it a try.

To my surprise, the notes went together creating an unusual, yet aesthetic, combination of notes and tones. The first release was not meditative, relaxing music nor was it supposed to be. It was designed as a pathogen-killing set of frequencies. My wife and I, along with others, have found relief from colds, sinus irritations and sore throat symptoms. In real-life, the frequencies were experimentally used to reverse diagnosed swine flu symptoms that were resistant to Tamiflu.

The second release I created based on Sharry's finding contains the original eight-minute Swine Flu (Le Ciel The Sky) frequency set that has been combined with relaxing meditation sounds. The result is a 30-minute sound journey, called Sines of Life: Arrival of Healing that is designed to relax the body into a state of self-healing.

Can these results be trusted? Many years of research substantiate the ability of music and sound to support optimal human form and function. What more can you ask for?

Do these techniques conform to the standards of conventional medical practice? No, but you cannot argue with the results.

How does it work?

I don't think any of us can answer that yet. We only know that it does and that the public has a right to know about it.

In my case, standard medical practice had nothing to offer. I was told to go home and die. I believe that frequency-based biomarkers that can be translated into sound and music holds the potential to change the face of medicine. This is 'Star Trek' medicine brought to life NOW by a very dedicated woman with very unusual talents that can benefit the world of medicine and self healing. This may be too new, too innovative, too "out there" for some people to wrap their heads around, but I'm living proof that it is real. For me it was literally a matter of life or death, and it saved my life. It can potentially help thousands of people who have been left with no conventional options.

In addition to being an acclaimed movie and television actor, James Marshall is a talented composer and musician. To learn more about his journey back to health working with Sharry Edwards, and to listen to and learn more about the Le Ciel compositions James has composed based on Sharry Edwards' research, visit www.bioacousticsolutions.net/le-ciel.

CHAPTER 1

HUMAN BIOACOUSTICS THERAPY— THE MEDICINE OF THE FUTURE IS ALREADY HERE

I magine this:

Wanting to know about your current health status, you speak into your cell phone, tablet, or computer to record your voice, speaking in normal tones for approximately 30 seconds.

Then, within minutes, after your voiceprint is analyzed by a proprietary software program, you receive an in-depth BioAcoustics-based report that comprehensively reveals your current nutritional status and needs—including any nutrient deficiencies, excesses, and other nutritional imbalances you have—as well as the health status of every major organ in your body, as well as an assessment of your current mental and emotional state and any potential psychological traits that may require your attention.

Because you are skeptical (and rightly so), with your results in hand, you immediately have your doctor screen you by ordering comprehensive blood and saliva panels, plus an urinalysis. When the results of these tests come back 24-48 hours later, both you and your doctor are surprised to discover that not only do they confirm the findings that the assessment of your voiceprint analysis provided, but that the voiceprint analysis also discovered additional concerns that your doctor's tests failed to uncover. These important discoveries are due to math-based protocols that analyze your voiceprint 16 layers deep.

Convinced of the value and accuracy of your voiceprint analysis, you then begin to use a tone box that plays sound frequencies specially prepared for your unique, individualized health needs, listening to them under headphones for 30 minutes twice a day. One month later, both you and your doctor are surprised by how much your health and overall emotional demeanor have improved, simply by listening to your sound frequencies.

Now let's take this a step further:

Based on your own health improvements, you decide to learn how to provide this same amazing health approach in order to offer it to your friends and family, and maybe even to others in your local community, and before long you are recognized by all those you help as a sound therapy provider as a true asset to everyone you serve.

Does this seem like utopian science fiction to you?

It isn't.

Not only are people all around the world gaining the same health benefits outlined above using these sound healing methods, many of them have also undergone training in these methods to help others. And in many cases, they have been doing this for years, all thanks to the pioneering discoveries I've made as the founder of the diagnostic and therapeutic modality called Human BioAcoustics™. In the pages that follow, I will teach you how it works, how it can improve your health, and how, if you are interested, you too can become a Human BioAcoustics practitioner. (My dream is to have at least one such practitioner in every town and city across the United States and beyond.)

An Example Of What Is Possible With Human BioAcoustics

You read about the dramatic recovery James Marshall was able to achieve by working with me. In Chapter 5, you will read about more remarkable results produced by Human BioAcoustics and the Vocal Profiling system of analysis and diagnostics that I developed. What follows is another example of how precisely this technology can work, one that illustrates how it is capable of detecting the different underlying causes of the same condition people are suffering from.

Years ago, I sent a letter to some of the doctors that I've worked with, informing them that I was conducting a project involving gait. I asked them to send me clients who had problems walking.

In the first week, I examined three people. The first was an older gentleman in his late 70's who was not walking well at all, and who had terrible difficulty turning around. He came in with his doctor and his wife, and, using Vocal Profiling, I found that he could not process vitamin B12, and that his levels of cobalt, which is contained in B12, were elevated eight times higher than normal. I had never heard of B12 causing someone's gait to be unstable, but that's exactly what was happening with this man. This was subsequently verified in a lab test.

By playing the Frequency Equivalent for B12, I was able to have him running up and down the yard in a couple of hours by himself. I don't want to take credit here; his body did the healing once the sound frequencies were introduced. In fact, I found the computer analysis questionable but I tried it anyway. Within hours of listening to the sounds he was able to walk briskly across the yard by himself.

The second person I worked with was a young lady who was knock-kneed and pigeon-toed, and she also had trouble with her gait. It turned out that her condition was due to the gene for Frederick's ataxia (FA), which I confirmed using Vocal Profiling. FA is a rare, inherited condition known to cause damage of the nervous system, muscle weakness, balance issues, and other problems. It is considered to be incurable and worsens over time. Unfortunately, though I thought I might be able to help her, at least to some degree, she refused my help.

The third client I worked with was man who was paralyzed in one leg and who didn't have very much use of the other. I was able to trace the cause of his paralysis down to a trauma to his L2 vertebra caused by a skiing accident. He didn't report that to us, but my technology was able to pinpoint that there was something very seriously wrong with his L2. When I explained this to him, he told me about his skiing accident. Once he received the proper sound frequencies, he was able to lay on his back and do bicycle kicks before he left that day, using both of his legs, something he hadn't been able to do in years.

These case histories are clear examples of how people with the same condition can have completely different causes for that condition. All three people had gait problems, but in the first person's case it was due to a biochemical imbalance, in the second it was genetic fault, and in the third it was due to a structural trauma. This illustrates why it's incredibly important to individualize people's medical care. Being able to do that is one of Human BioAcoustics' strong points. By using it, not only can we determine the causes for problems that have already arisen in people, but we can also evaluate factors that are predictive of what is going to happen to a person, and, most importantly, use the indicated sound frequencies that Vocal Profiling reveals preventively to avoid that.

How I Came To Develop Human BioAcoustics

I began my research into sound frequencies and healing over four decades ago, when audiological tests revealed that I was born with the unique ability to hear sounds beyond the normal range of human hearing, and that I am also able to vocally produce sine waves. In my first research project, testing showed that by the use of my voice I was able to control a person's blood pressure by as much as 32 points. Since then, through the concept of vocal coherence, I've demonstrated that the human voice is a unique frequency representation of the body's structural and biochemical status, and that, through the use of the voice spectral analysis techniques I've developed, the body is capable of diagnosing and prescribing for itself.

Recognizing the potential of my innate healing abilities, in 1982, I developed the BioAcoustics technology that enables others to mechanically reproduce the diagnostic and therapeutic results I have achieved. To date, thousands of health care practitioners have trained and been certified in my methods, which continue to garner serious attention from conventional health care facilities and HMO's worldwide. In October 2001, the International Association of New Science, bestowed its Scientist of the Year award to me in recognition of my work with BioAcoustics.

What Is Human BioAcoustics?: First of all, let me say that the work I am doing is in Human BioAcoustics. There is also a field of animal BioAcoustics which has been around for a long time. There's a research center at Cornell University, for example, that is involved in this, and others in Texas and England. Researchers in this field analyze the sounds animals emit to determine their health, and it can also to tell where the animals are from. Birds from the south, even though they are the same species, sound a little different from birds of the north, for example. At the time I began my work, I didn't even know the term *bioacoustics* existed; I thought I'd made it up.

BioAcoustics means "life sounds", and as I use the term, it describes the field of research involving the use of voice spectral analysis (Vocal Profiling) and low frequency sound to help the body reverse its own disease. It can most aptly be described as a cross between music therapy and biofeedback. It is related to music therapy in the sense that certain sounds are used to stimulate the healing process, although not necessarily sounds that are considered musical. And it is related to biofeedback in that, as these low frequency sounds are presented to the person, they elicit specific biological and emotional responses.

I should point out that Human BioAcoustics is not to be confused with what is known as frequency therapy, which uses ranges that are not considered to be auditory and is delivered through transducers placed on the body. Nor is it the same thing as music therapy, because the sounds used are not always within the range of vocal or instrumental octaves. Human BioAcoustics uses low frequency ambient sounds which can be delivered to the client in a sound chamber, through speakers, or through headphones.

There are two distinct processes to Human BioAcoustics, both of which are essential if maximum results are to be achieved. The first process involves determining the individual vocal patterns of the person, which is done before any sound frequencies are presented. This process is called BioAcoustic Vocal Profiling. Once the person's vocal pattern has been determined, sets of sound formulas are specifically created and presented to that person, which are designed to positively influence and integrate the systems within the body that produce, interpret, and otherwise use frequency. My research has found that, for health to be present, the body requires the presence of a full spectrum of harmonious frequencies working together cooperatively. In a very real sense, you can liken the body as a musical instrument. When it is out of tune, the result is discordant, but when the instrument is tuned, the sounds become consonant.

The idea of using sound to facilitate change within the body is not new. Almost every culture throughout recorded history has used sound and movement to influence mood. For thousands of years, practitioners of Tibetan medicine have known of the positive vibrational effects of bells and chanting, for instance, and ancient philosophers such as Pythagoras, Plato, and Aristotle taught that the human body reflects the sounds and tones that exist within its personal environment. And, of course, in the Bible we are told that, "In the beginning was the Word," and that through the agency of that Word all of creation came into being. In other words, frequency is the basis of our universe. It wasn't until recently, however, that computerized technology and instrumentation advanced to the stage where we are now able to use this technology to use sound frequencies diagnostically and therapeutically to literally create "sound health".

The term "sound health" is actually a play on words. I think that we've known about the relationship between sound and health all along, but we were able to deal with it in our language much quicker than we've been able to deal with it as a technology or an idea related to well-being.

For instance, when my husband and I go to the grocery store and he picks up a grapefruit to see if it's ripe, I listen to it, and if it has a clear note of E, I know it is a nice, fresh grapefruit and I'll say, "It sounds good to me."

This is an expression that people have always used to convey their perception that something is right or "sound." This also shows up in phrases like "sound advice," and so forth. Sound means "stable" or "foundational," and it also refers to frequency and music. And there is a feedback loop between the sounds that people make and the sounds that people hear. It's the only dual feedback loop that is like that in the body. You don't make color with your eyes, for example, but you do use your eyes to perceive color.

When I say the grapefruit sounds good to me, most people automatically think I mean that buying the grapefruit sounds like a good idea, but I literally mean that it sounds like a good grapefruit. This has always been an innate ability in me, and for many years it didn't occur to me other people didn't have it. I have always been able to tell what was going on with people by the sound of their voice. For instance, when I was young I noticed that my aunt had a sound that was new to her, and that it was the same sound that my grandmother had when she had diabetes. So I thought that maybe my aunt had diabetes too, and it turned out that she did.

I really think my ability is a trait that we forgot or have literally tuned out of our sensory repertoire. When you read some of the ancient literature about Socrates, Pythagoras, and people like that, you find that they heard these sounds, as well. I hear sounds from nearly everything. I cannot hear sounds from plastic, but I hear sounds from everything else—animals, trees and flowers. And I decided to use my ability as a means of helping others to experience better health, using BioAcoustics to make the diagnostic and therapeutic elements of health care more precise.

We already do something similar with cars. We can take our cars into the garage and plug them in and have a machine evaluate exactly what's wrong, but with conventional medicine, we don't have that ability in relation to our own bodies. We have CT scans, MRIs and X-rays, and other devices that we've created, but these are not diagnostic enough to individuate for each of us. When we evaluate people via frequency, we find that their bone and their muscle structure are pretty nearly the same, but when it comes to the body's organs we start to become very individual. We're all singing the same song when it comes to our structure, but when it comes to our organs we're singing a slightly different tune. And when you come to emotions, we each create our own scale, not just our own song.

Let me tell you a bit more about how I got involved in this. As I mentioned, I was born with my ability to hear the sounds emitted by the body, and at first I just took it for granted that everybody could hear these sounds. Later on, of course, I realized that wasn't true. Then, when I was in college and typing a paper for one of my professors on tinnitus, I read that hearing these kinds of sounds was an illness. So I went to have my hearing tested. It turned out that not only could I hear just fine, but that I also hear sound well beyond the normal range of human hearing, and that I can vocally reproduce these sounds in the form of sine waves. I did this with the man who was administering my hearing test, and when I sang his tones he reported that his blood pressure decreased.

He was very interested in that result for a couple of reasons. One, he was aware that Samurai warriors used to yell right before they attacked an opponent to decrease their blood pressure so they would have a split second of advantage. Two, he was a young man and wanted to start a family, but the high blood pressure medication he was on was rendering him impotent, so he was very interested to see if, through sounds, we could help him with his blood pressure issue.

This was the first research project that I was involved in. It was a pilot study and from it we found that by using my voice we could reduce blood pressure levels by as much as 32 points. From there, the research snowballed. I would listen to a person's sound and then vocally reproduce it onto a recording and take it back to the laboratory to see what it revealed on a spectrograph. From this, I could determine what frequencies were too high or too low in the voice, and I found that there was little to no vocal coherence in somebody who was ill.

When there are gaps in the measurements and things that are too high or too low, then we know that the person has some unbalance by way of his frequencies in the body. But I knew that if this could only be done by me because of my abilities, then we were very limited. This led me to search for a way to replicate my abilities through technology without me having to be present. By this time, I knew that the sounds I was hearing were being emitted from people's ears, but when I talked to my professors of speech and hearing, I was told, "Sharry please, there is nothing in the ear that creates a sound." But a few years later Dr. Wendell Browne, of Johns Hopkins University, published some papers about otoacoustic emissions, which proved that there really was sound coming out of the ear. And here we were doing all of this work under the assumption that this was something esoteric in my ears alone. Now I can teach almost anyone to hear their own sound if they're not deaf. I show you how in Chapter 2.

As I continued my research, I eventually discovered what I was looking for and had computerized instrumentation built that can enable anyone, with proper training, to do what I do. Many people have now received the training and use the equipment. About half of them are medical practitioners, and the rest are caretakers for family members or other people suffering from chronic disease. Instead of them having to return to us time and time again, we're able to train them to take this out into the world. In exchange, we ask that they share with us the data they are collecting, since we are essentially an educational research center.

What Happens During A Human BioAcoustics Session

A session begins with the person speaking into a special microphone that we originally designed. The gives us a recording of the governing patterns of what I called their Signature Sound. This is entered into a computer, which then does what is called a Fast Fourier Transform and creates a computerized representation of the voice, decibel, and frequency, as well as the architecture of the voice itself, by way of the shape of the wave form. We then evaluate the reading to see what points are too high or too low. Points that are located high on the graph, called "risers," indicate sound frequencies that are loud and overabundant, while points that are low, known as "stringers," indicate frequencies that are not as readily apparent. The objective is to create a smaller, more unified pattern of fewer risers and/or stringers, which is an indication of more coherence.

The frequencies that are lacking, overabundant, or dissident can then be used to construct sets of frequency formulations that people can use to help them reverse whatever imbalances may be present. For example, our research has shown that adults and children who have been diagnosed with so-called attention deficit disorder have the Frequency Equivalent of adrenaline that is way too high, meaning that it's in the body and it can't be used. When we give them the Frequency Equivalent of adrenaline and they start using adrenaline it calms them down, because the frequency allows the body to identify the compound and use it appropriately.

What we have found is that when people have risers that are too high, it means that there is either a toxin in the body, or some other compound that the body doesn't know how to use because it doesn't recognize it. Stress, man-made electricity, being around machinery, and these kinds of things causes our frequencies to drop out or to become over-abundant, and as we examine the vocal spectral analysis and find out what's too high or too low, or what's missing or thin in the voice, we can tell what's going on bioacoustically with someone's health.

Once we have that information, we know what frequencies the person needs. We have a little box that is like a miniature computer into which we download the frequencies. You hook it up to a speaker and turn it on and listen to the frequencies just as you would listen to music, or you can listen to it with headphones.

The reason that Human BioAcoustics is delivered to the client via headphones is for protection. This technology is very powerful, and the frequencies that are used are specific to the needs of the client. But just as a healthy physician can become sick or develop side-effects if he takes medications intended for his sick patients, so can other people, including the BioAcoustics provider, be negatively affected if they listen to sound frequencies not intended for them. This is something people need to be very aware of. The potential of frequency is tremendous and you can't just apply it willy-nilly and expect good and safe results.

The results people achieve depends on their condition. Depending on their symptoms, treatment can be either short- or long-term. In most cases, reassessment, monitoring, and program adjustment are essential for continued improvement. But one of the big advantages of Human BioAcoustics, as the gait examples I shared above illustrate, is that a person's symptoms that are often conflicting can be separated and identified using Vocal Profiling, including in cases where conventional evaluation is unable to determine the underlying cause. In the case of the man with the vitamin B12 problems, for instance, he had originally been diagnosed at the Mayo Clinic as having peripheral neuropathy, which actually turned out not to be the case at all.

Another advantage of Human BioAcoustics is that it acts as an ideal complement or adjunct to other therapies, both diagnostically and therapeutically. In addition, what we are finding is that the diagnosis in and of itself is not as important as identifying and introducing the indigenous frequencies of the person's originating patterns. The diagnosis of digestive upset, for example, is not as important as presenting the frequency that will enhance or resolve a person's specific digestive difficulties.

I need to emphasize, however, that a person's outcome using Human BioAcoustics is in large part due to his or her willingness to follow the protocol prescribed by the practitioner. Each person is evaluated on an individual basis, and each protocol is designed specifically for that person. The most common frustration I have in this regard is convincing the client to continue listening to the frequencies after he or she begins to experience improvement. This is similar to a physician's frustration when a patient stops using antibiotics once he starts feeling better, and then his infection comes back. I've had a number of clients who came back to me embarrassed because their symptoms had returned and it turned out they hadn't been following their protocol. Therefore, I tell the people I train as Human BioAcoustics providers that it is essential that they take an active role in supervising each case, to ensure that their clients use this technology in the way that the providers suggest.

One other thing I'd like to mention is the placebo effect. We've had skeptics try to dismiss the results we've achieved by saying the person got better because he or she expected to, not because Human BioAcoustics actually works. While I firmly believe in the power of the mind to influence healing, the outcomes Human BioAcoustics has achieved are verified by a variety of diagnostic tests and measurements and, in many cases, follow-up evaluations by our clients' physicians. In addition, we have had many cases that have shown improvement among people who had little or no awareness about what is expected, including newborns and persons who were comatose.

Decloaking and Addressing Pathogens To Speed Healing of Infectious Disease

Throughout history, mankind has been plagued by infectious diseases. With the advent of modern biochemical antibiotics, many of these older diseases seem to have been eradicated. However, many new diseases have been identified, some of which are mutations of previously "cured" diseases, in the form of resistant pathogens. Antibiotic-resistant bacteria are a well-known example of this.

Our entire ecosystem has now become vulnerable to these resistant pathogens due to the fact that, as these invaders move from host to host, they mutate, to the point where what worked against them in the past may no longer work today. This has caused extreme concern for those in charge of public health. If we don't have the resources to keep up with the mutations, how can the public be protected? How will the people even know how to take precautions against infection?

Controversial biophysicist Hulda Clark, PhD, ND (October 18, 1928 – September 3 2009), stated in her book, *The Cure For All Disease*, that cancer, one of the most feared of diseases, is caused by pathogens—specifically, parasites whose life cycles are aided and abetted by the modern chemicals that we encounter in our environment. Clark was certainly not alone in identifying links between parasites/pathogens and modern illness. Researchers have found that chronic fatigue syndrome (CFS) shows a strong connection with Epstein Barr virus, for example, and that *Chlamydia pneumoniae* is often a causative factor in heart disease and pulmonary embolism. The list of pathogens and their connection to many disease is long and growing.

To add to the problem, these pathogens are able to use the body's processes against it. Using the sloughed-off protein of the host, these pathogens have the ability to create a protective cloak so that the body will be fooled into thinking that the pathogen is part of our normal form and function.

What can be done to combat this problem? In seeking to answer that question, I conducted studies using Human BioAcoustics. I wanted to find a way to look at the cloaking mechanism of pathogens, because I knew that invading pathogens make use of leftover protein debris in the body to create a coating that prevents the body's defense systems from recognizing them as something foreign. I wanted to find a way to look at the pathogens and destroy the protein barrier, and I found we were able to do this using specific frequencies. To do this requires different kinds of frequencies for different kinds of pathogens.

The frequency for the Epstein Barr virus, for instance, is very different from the frequency for yeast or Streptococcus. Each pathogen has its own frequency and it buries itself inside this protein debris to cloak itself, so that even if there is a neutrophil right beside it that should recognize and attack the pathogen as a foreign substance, it doesn't. This is one of the ways that disease takes hold in the body. But when you begin to decloak the pathogen by using the proper sound frequency, the body's defense system of antigens, neutrophils, natural killer cells, and so forth come in and start to devour it.

I demonstrated this years ago with a pilot study involving 17 participants in which the Epstein Barr virus, yeast, and the *Chlamydia pneumoniae* bacterium were targeted, and in each case Human BioAcoustics successfully eradicated these conditions by decloaking the protein coating that cloaked them from the body's immune agents. This was confirmed by darkfield microscopy [analysis of live blood cells] and conventional lab testing. What I discovered was that Human BioAcoustics technology, as has been shown under microscopic observation, is able to dissolve the ringed protein barrier used by some of these pathogens to cloak themselves.

In my initial studies, the technique was used successfully against the Epstein Barr virus, *Chlamydia pneumoniae bacterium* and yeast.

At the beginning of the studies, frequencies identified in Dr Clark's book were used, but I found that these were not accurate or that mutations in the pathogens had taken place, thus making these frequencies unusable and necessitating the search for new, correct frequencies.

Below is a short review of the initial study in which the Epstein Barr virus, the Chlamydia pneumoniae bacterium and yeast were targeted. (Note that in the case of the yeast, the decloaking and deactivation happened so quickly that the yeast could not be seen within a minute or so.)

Epstein Barr Virus: A filmed recording of the activity under the microscope showed that when the coating of the Epstein Barr virus was dissolved, the neutrophils (the white blood cells that attack invaders) were activated. The activity of the neutrophils was nil until the Epstein Barr was decloaked by the appropriate frequency, even though the two were only separated by minute distances. As the decloaking transpired, it was obvious that the neutrophil had not been aware of the invader until the protein coating had begun to dissolve. After the decloaking, the neutrophil continued to consume the invading pathogen.

Here are some additional notes from the study:

- This is listed by Dr Clark as having the musical note of C#, but we found it to range from mid C# to early D.
- When the pathogen numbers were high, there was an active invasion as well as symptoms (the most common being fatigue) which varied in intensity.
- When the antigen frequencies were high, antibodies were being produced.

- When detoxing the Epstein Barr virus, ear and throat infections, pain and sensitivity in those areas were noticed. Reports show that Epstein Barr virus tends to hide in the neck area.

Chlamydia pneumoniae: Human BioAcoustic voice spectral analysis has been shown to be an inexpensive (conventional lab testing for Chlamydia pneumoniae can cost hundreds of dollars per test) and quick way to determine which pathogens are present and which antibodies have been manufactured by the body. In the case of Chlamydia pneumoniae, we were able to identify those participants in the study who had been infected by the bacterium, those who had created antibodies to it, and those who were on their way to being free of the infection.

Additional notes from the study are as follows:

- This bacterium was not listed by Dr Clark.
- This is not the sexually transmitted variety of Chlamydia; the Chlamydia pneumoniae strain is airborne and it attacks the lungs and pulmonary system. Its symptoms include labored breathing, dizziness and passing out, accelerated heart rate, high blood pressure and muddled thinking. Re-infection is possible after symptoms have disappeared. The bacterium has an incubation period of 10–14 days.
- The frequency of Chlamydia pneumoniae corresponds with the musical note of C#, and also involves the note of A, which is associated with blood clotting.
- For active cases, a narrow band of C# was active in each chart, and late A to early A# was also involved. For those with high protease levels, symptoms did not appear.
- For those with blood type O, symptoms were short and less severe.
- When the Frequency Equivalent™ of Epstein Barr virus was high, an active infection was present.
- When the antigen frequencies were high, antibodies were being produced.

- The Chlamydia pneumoniae formed clots which formed a protective coating that cloaked the entire clot from the neutrophils. These clots are not shown in chest X-rays or clotting factor scans. It is suggested that a pulmonary arteriography or a spiral CT of the lung be ordered to verify the presence of these small clots in the lung tissue.

- Eating fatty foods or heavy meals exacerbated symptoms of labored breathing. Depending on how much fatty food or how large the meal had been consumed by the participant, symptoms would dissipate within half an hour to four hours after sound presentation. Participants who had poor digestion of protein were most vulnerable. Improving protein (including milk protein) digestion is a major step in eliminating the availability of sloughed-off protein that is used for cloaking by such pathogens as Chlamydia pneumoniae.

- Doxycycl HYC, a potent antibiotic, is reported to be able to kill this strain of Chlamydia pneumoniae, but had little effect in this case. Giving the frequency equivalent for Doxycycl produced side effects as if the medication had been given, even though the subject had never taken it before.

- One infected and particularly vulnerable client exhibited small, thin, pinch-like bruises.

- One client had a pacemaker implanted by doctors, to stop an accelerated heart rate, but the breathing problems and muddled thinking were still present after the placement of the pacemaker.

- One client was told that he needed heart surgery to clear blocked arteries, but, obtaining a second opinion, he discovered that this was not necessary.

- One client was told by the medical establishment that absolutely nothing was wrong, except simply stress.

- Four persons in the study ended up in the hospital, but not one hospital discovered that a pathogen was causing the problem.

Another example of the ability of Human BioAcoustics to decloak pathogens and resolve infectious diseases involved a woman who came to me who was suffering with severe fatigue and lack of energy. Her medical tests provided little help in resolving her condition, but a darkfield blood examination revealed that Laura had Epstein Barr virus. The frequencies of Epstein Barr also showed up as an invading pathogen in my analysis of her vocal print.

A mathematical set of formulas was developed and used to decloak the pathogen and assist the body to identify the intruder. Once the pathogen was pointed out, the killer cells of the body easily identified and attacked the pathogen. This also worked well with the bacteria and yeast overgrowth her vocal print revealed in her body. Soon, she was no longer fatigued and resumed her active lifestyle.

Using frequency to decloak these pathogens is the first step in establishing control over them. Royal Rife and many others knew that frequency is the key to controlling pathogens. It is the key to stimulating the body to fight its own pathogens. The main issue has been finding the correct frequency, in light of the pathogens' constant mutations, and the appropriate wave form.

Giving the body direct square waves can cause damage. The new techniques must provide frequencies in exacting patterns, using short bursts, for approximately eight minutes. Using frequency in this way provides a very powerful and effective avenue to dissolve the ringed protein barriers. This is indicative of the potential Human BioAcoustics has for detecting and eradicating a wide range of pathogenic disease agents.

The sound formulas must always be determined on a case-by-case basis. This is very important to understand. The same is true with people who have the same symptoms of infectious agent. Each person is unique and will respond to the sounds in his or her unique fashion. To determine the most effective frequencies, in all cases it is first necessary to employ vocal spectral analysis, and then proceed based on what the person's vocal profile reveals. In some cases, a very narrow frequency range is required to achieve the desired effect; in others, a broader range of frequencies may be more appropriate.

Why does frequency work to dissolve ringed protein barriers used by resistant pathogens to cloak themselves? And what is frequency?

Light is frequency. Sound is frequency. Aroma is frequency. Emotion is frequency. Vibration is frequency. Music is frequency. Brain waves are frequency. Nerve impulses are frequency. Everything, at its most common denominator, is frequency. Frequency is everything and everything is frequency. In reality, there are no solids. We exist in a universe that consists entirely of energy. Einstein proved this. Frequency defines it.

How does the body know what to do with all of these frequencies? The body hears frequency. The ears change that sensory input into biochemical impulses and send that information to the brain. The eyes feast on frequencies of light input, change those impulses into biochemical energy and send that information to the brain. The nose receives aromas. Each impulse is changed into biochemical input and sent to the brain. Each sensory organ collects information as frequency input and changes that input into biochemical impulses which it sends to the brain. The brain in turn digitizes the information and redistributes it to systems and functions of the body so that the body can maintain homoeostasis.

How does the brain know how to route these inputs to the appropriate part of the brain? Answer: by the octave of frequency. If the frequency comes in at a level of:

- 1–2 cycles per second, the brain interprets this as biomagnetic input;
- 2–4 cycles per second, the brain interprets this as bioelectrical input;
- 1–4 cycles per second, the brain interprets this as genetic frequency input (biomagnetic and bioelectric input combined);
- 4–8 cycles per second, the brain interprets this as biochemical input;

- 8–16 cycles per second, the brain interprets this as structural (muscular/skeletal) input;
- 16–32 cycles per second, the brain interprets this as neurophysical input.

Each frequency, or frequency set, has specific functions, both structural and functional, within the body. Each frequency set does its own work and can share frequencies from its set for other biological systems to use. This has been known to occur but, until recently, the mechanism by which it occurred was not defined.

The body, in its infinite wisdom, has a perfect feedback loop to make it possible for the body to diagnose and provide a set of healing frequencies as a self-diagnosis and prescription. The system—the voice to provide sound, and the ear to perceive sound—is a perfect diagnostic tool that can provide reliable predictive, preventive and curative options for self-healing. In no other system in the body is a feedback loop used in such a conscious way. This system is operating even when we are comatose. It only ceases when our life-force ceases—and we really don't know that for sure. Our ears transmit a stabilizing sound, an oto-acoustic emission, which is a constant attempt to provide healing frequencies to the body.

This ability is now being considered as a viable complement to modern medicine, but references from ancient civilizations reveal that sound had been used for thousands of years to balance and maintain health. Tibetans know the positive vibrational effects of bells and chanting. Traditional Chinese medicine practitioners recognize that properly flowing energy, or chi, is fundamental to good, balanced health. The Bible equates "the Word", a form of sound, with God and creation.

Today it seems that these ancient wisdoms are being revisited as conventional medicine, with its previous reliance upon the scientific method, begins to pay attention to the potential of frequency to nourish and support the body's capacity to self-heal.

Other Health Issues That Can Be Addressed By Human Bioacoustics Technology

My research is ongoing and I continue to make new discoveries about the potential Human BioAcoustics has to offer, not only in terms of health, but for other issues, as well. To date the frequency formulas based on people's Signature Sounds have been able to assist the healing process for a wide range of structural, neurological, and biochemical conditions. These include identifying pathogens, biochemical toxins, and genetic syndromes, and diagnostically and therapeutically addressing a wide range of health conditions, including muscle stress and weakness, nutritional imbalances, attention problems and learning disorders, environmental allergies, arthritis, emphysema, epilepsy, heart disease, cerebral palsy, chronic pain, osteoporosis, blood sugar problems, metabolic disorders (including obesity), gout, and sports injuries.

Working with muscle has actually been one of the easiest areas in which to see the benefits that Human BioAcoustics can provide, because there is such immediate feedback from the musculature itself. We are able to take a vocal print and then use it to determine what muscles are going to be weak or strong, or which ones are already weak or strong, and to what degree. We then present low frequency sound that will change the muscle strength. We've shown this in double-blind studies.

Think about the applications this has. Take sports injuries, for instance. We'll be able to look at them before they happen. Nursing homes is another area. We can actually exercise the muscles of people in old age without them ever moving, simply by applying the proper sound frequencies. And for people who have operations and are cut over a muscle, we can begin to exercise that while they're still under anesthesia. Assisting the recovery from surgery and other issues, like macular degeneration, is an example of this. We've already done that a number of times.

And think of how this could work in exercise clubs. We could take a person's vocal print and tell people what you need to work on each day, according to which of their muscles that day are shown to be weak or strong. We can do this for all muscles at the same time, which is something that an exercise physiologist would have trouble pinpointing until a problem actually occurred.

Another area where we are having a high degree of success is in the resolution of gout. Gout can be an extremely debilitating condition, and it affects over six million people a year, according to the National Arthritis Foundation. In addition, there is no reliable test for gout, nor are flare-ups predictable, and the side-effects caused by conventional medications used to treat it can be severe, including, in some cases, serious interference in bone marrow function. So I decided to see if Human BioAcoustics would have any benefit in this area, and what I discovered is that specific low frequency sound was able to positively alleviate the stress of gout pain in approximately 90 percent of the people I worked with. Further independent studies and observations by two physicians confirmed the results.

My work in this area led to the development of the G-OUT Out tone generator, a small, portable device that gout sufferers can use.

As I mentioned, one of the significant values that Human BioAcoustics has is that it can be used predictively to assess a person's health status, including before health symptoms become apparent. As an example of this, I once had a visit from a man who had heard about the work I was doing and he was curious to see if BioAcoustics could reveal in this regard. I agreed to analyze his voice, and his vocal print indicated that he had a serious thyroid condition. This came as a complete surprise to him since he had no history or medical evidence of such a problem. To verify my findings, he went to see his physician, but the lab tests he received indicated nothing abnormal. So both he and his doctor had a good laugh about the worthlessness of my analysis and he went about his business.

A few days later, he collapsed due to a series of mysterious symptoms that stumped the medical professionals who treated him. His heartbeat was erratic, he was sweating profusely, and he was anxious and disoriented, but they were unable to determine why. Then he remember my analysis and suggested they take a look at his thyroid. This time, tests showed that he did indeed have a serious thyroid problem that was causing his symptoms: a thyroid storm, a rare but severe and life-threatening complication of hyperthyroidism. The vocal print had revealed he was at risk for this nine days earlier.

Another example of this involved a seven-year-old girl who found herself unable to read in school. The year before, she was a top reader in her class, but suddenly she couldn't read anymore. Things got so bad that she was put into a special remedial reading class. This embarrassed Andi and made her reluctant to go to school. She cried every day. On the days she didn't cry, she pretended to be sick. Eventually her mother brought her to see me.

Vocal testing was used to determine if there were any biochemical reasons for the girl's reading problems. During that session, while she was receiving low-frequency sound, she was able to read clearly and without hesitation. The test pointed to the possibility that she had been poisoned by formaldehyde, a chemical preservative.

A detoxification program was initiated, and her teacher noticed immediate and striking differences in the girl. Her self-esteem soared. She was again a bright, cheerful, intelligent child she had been before the poisoning occurred. Best of all, she could read again.

An example that illustrates the value Human BioAcoustics has both diagnostically and therapeutically involved a woman who had Paget's disease, a chronic condition that causes enlarged and weakened bones. Her condition left her bones light and porous and in a constant state of destruction. She came to me on crutches after breaking her hip and being released from the hospital.

Because Paget's disease is considered incurable, her physician expected that her condition would continue to worsen as her bones further deteriorated. In her first session with me, analysis of her voice revealed that her body was deficient in a specific nutrient mineral. I won't say what it is, because I don't want people to think that all they have to do to treat Paget's disease is take a nutrient, but in this woman's case, once the nutrient was added to her daily intake of vitamins, she began to improve and eventually no longer needed her crutches. In fact, a few months later, she called to tell me she had been out square dancing, which never would have been possible had my analysis of her vocal profile not discovered the nutrient she needed.

I've already told you about Human BioAcoustics' value in the area of muscle stress and trauma, but let me share one final example with you. One of our local attorneys was an avid tennis player, but some years ago he injured his leg in a motorcycle accident—so severely, that his doctors wanted to amputate. He refused this, but after years of physical therapy, he was told that there was no hope that he would ever again walk normally. The lower portion of his leg was as large as a football; he could not walk straight, nor bend his ankle, and he'd lost all stamina for exercise. Eventually, he was forced to close his law practice and wound up living with his parents. That's when he found out about the work I was doing.

Within two months of regular Human BioAcoustics' sessions, he not only could once again walk straight, he was back on the tennis court and was playing so well that he was asked to be the tennis coach at the local high school.

Harmonious Health

These examples represent only a small part of the benefits Human BioAcoustics holds as a healing therapy. While it is certainly not a cure-all, our inventory of unsuccessful outcomes is short. Human BioAcoustics is most appropriate for nonemergency health conditions, on a predictive, diagnostic, and/or therapeutic basis. But I do not recommend it for emergency situations, such as poisoning, traumatic bleeding, broken bones, or situations like heart attack or appendicitis. I would never recommend that it be used to set a broken bone, for example, but I would not hesitate to offer it to accelerate healing, reduce pain and swelling, and reduce the recuperation time of such an accident.

The field of vocal analysis, utilizing the idea that frequencies contained in the voice are holographic representations of one's state of health, is quickly gaining a reputation for excellence.

Research has repeatedly shown that every muscle, compound, process and structure of the body has a frequency equivalent that can be mathematically calculated. This provides the foundation for the concept that the body's ability to heal itself can originate as frequency interactions between the molecular signals of the entire body. When these patterns become discordant, dis-ease is the result. When presented the correct low-frequency analog sound, a new harmony can result, with the person experiencing notable self-healing.

The Potential Future of Human Bioacoustics

Interest in Human BioAcoustics is definitely growing, especially among the health practitioners who are finding out about it. At the same time, however, many practitioners and organizations are hesitant to explore BioAcoustics because it isn't approved by the Food and Drug Administration (FDA) or the American Medical Association, and organizations like that. I had one doctor contact me, for instance, who was very interested in the work I am doing with gout. He asked to see any double-blind studies I had on this. I don't have any to offer him, because when I contacted the National Institutes of Health to inform them of what I was doing, they told me that the best way to facilitate its efficacy was through the collection and documentation of case studies, which is what I've done. But when I told the doctor this, he said he couldn't get involved without double-blind studies because it would mean setting himself up to be sued. And he's right.

I think anybody who is bringing in a new paradigm should expect some resistance. I think it would be a sorry world if everything anybody said was automatically accepted. A certain amount of skepticism is needed to keep us on the path of doing the best we can. So it's up to me, the person who conceived and developed Human BioAcoustics, to educate people and find a way for them to accept its usefulness, and to do that I have to meet them where they are. Which is exactly why I've set up my educational research center and am training people to bring this out into the world. The more people we train and the more data we collect, the faster we can grow.

I think the promise of Human BioAcoustics in terms of health care will continue to grow. Right now, one of the biggest problems facing us as a nation is the exorbitant costs associated with health care. A significant part of these costs has to do with the ability to detect disease before it progresses to serious proportions. Human BioAcoustics has much to offer in this area, due to its effectiveness as a predictive and diagnostic tool.

Other areas of high medical costs include rehabilitation expenses, the side-effects of unsuitable medication, and long-term costs for lingering or incurable disease. These costs can also be ameliorated using Human BioAcoustics. For example, using voice spectral analysis, we have the ability to match medications or nutritional agents to a person's specific needs. We can do this with insulin for diabetes for, for instance. There are many different kinds of insulin, and right now finding the right form to use can be a process of trial and error, sometimes even requiring hospitalization until the proper form is found. We can determine what form to use by looking at which form best matches a person's vocal print.

Among the uses that I foresee for Human BioAcoustics are:

- Individualized, holistic, predictive and preventative health screening
- Drug and nutritional evaluation
- Nonintrusive blood chemistry screening
- Nonintrusive temperature control
- Depiction of disease root causes and disease pathways
- Identification of viral, bacterial, and fungal infections
- Identification of stress, paralyzed, or inactive muscles.

Among the areas of medicine that are most ready for a direct integration of Human BioAcoustics with conventional diagnostic and treatment methods are physical therapy, dietetics, physical therapy and massage, emergency medical technologies, and sports medicine. I also think it will prove to be of benefit during space travel, since we can use the frequency to exercise muscles during conditions of weightlessness.

Another area that I feel Human BioAcoustics could have much value is with future pandemics, and in addressing bioterrorism attacks from germ and biochemical warfare, which has now become a very serious challenge, as the recent COVID pandemic proved. Using voice spectral analysis, just as we have been able to identify and reverse infection due to pathogens such as the Epstein Barr virus, Streptococcus and *Chlamydia pneumoniae*, we can also identify the Frequency Equivalents™ for pathogens such as anthrax and smallpox. In addition, not only can the Frequency Equivalents of these pathogens be identified, but low frequency analog sound can be used to stimulate the body to eliminate them.

Ultimately, I would like to see Human BioAcoustics used in every facility that deals with people's health in any way, from hospitals, health clinics, and HMO's, to health clubs and health food stores. So that people everywhere could have the benefit of using it to determine what they need in order to achieve and maintain optimal health. Because it's a complete system that is very predictive, diagnostic, and therapeutic.

But I also want to stress that health care is only one area for which Human BioAcoustics holds great value. Now that the foundation work has been completed, I'm realizing that the possibilities for it are far more extensive than I once imagined.

Among the other areas for which preliminary research indicates that Human BioAcoustics is feasible are medical monitoring through voice spectral analysis over the telephone, the individuation of medications to reduce side-effect risk, drug and chemical screening for law enforcement agencies, immediate prediction of labor and delivery in cases of pregnancy, large area pest control without environmental side-effects, nontoxic fertilization, food preservation, and reversal of environmental pollution. The sky's the limit, really.

The Time Has Come To Make This Information Widely Known

When I first started to bring this work to the public, I met with a brilliant attorney named Naomi.

She warned me that this extraordinary information would be attacked from those who fear what I'm sharing and by those who wish to steal it from me. She advised me that I needed to think of a way to protect the information so that no one would actually understand the many layers of what they were dealing with.

At the same time, I was studying brain dominance as part of my undergraduate studies so I decided to present the entire body of the work from what I'm calling "right-brained convention." It is my belief that right- and left-brained persons perceive the universe differently, especially with regard to color. A left-brained person may perceive the frequencies assigned to the color red as red, while a right-brained person might actually be experiencing those frequencies as red's complementary color, green.

There is no way to prove this concept, but during my studies of frequency and brain dominance, I noticed that left- or right-brained persons wanted to receive frequencies differently. By describing my work the way, it has protected me from lazy thieves and overly critical academicians, and also from overly greedy financial institutions. It has protected me for many years, but as this is likely the last notable publication before I move on to the next dimension, it is time to lay a greater overview for Human BioAcoustics. Anyone could have figured out my protection strategy had they dared to look beyond the surface.

It is an honor to bring this information to the world's populace to help create a more prosperous future. That is why I wrote this book.

CHAPTER 2

EVERYBODY HAS A SIGNATURE SOUND

I magine a world in which we can be individually identified, manipulated and managed through the use of frequency-based biomarkers that can easily be obtained through our vocal sounds. That world already exists.

As you learned in Chapter 1, my development of Human BioAcoustics came about because of the ability I was born with to literally hear the sounds emitted by the human body, as well as those emitted by animals and plants. What I came to discover is that each of us possesses what I call the Signature Sound. This Signature Sound is the sonic frequency representation of all that you are.

The following example is a case in point: Russ Rudy, MD, had been diagnosed with multiple sclerosis (MS), resulting in serious leg muscle atrophy and neuropathy. Rudy was informed that his situation was dire, incurable and nothing more medically could be done for him. He was sent home to die with a Baclofen pump internally installed to help control his pain.

Instead of accepting this death sentence, Rudy came to see me, hopeful that I might be able to help him. I conducted a computerized evaluation of Rudy's vocal expressions (Vocal Profile), which identified biomarkers that indicated the presence of spinal damage and further indicated that no MS markers were present. Rudy denied that he had experienced any such physical trauma, but a few days later he remembered a skiing accident that had happened to him 20 years prior, which confirmed the computer identified spinal injury.

I then created specific ambient sound combinations designed to entrain Rudy's brain to return the body to normal form and function, based on the unique, individual properties of his voice. Over the next few weeks, lab reports confirmed that nerve recruitment was taking place from Rudy's waist to his toes. This is considered totally impossible by standard medical practice.

Before long, the Baclofen pump was removed (something that is usually only done at autopsy) because Rudy's legs now supported him and he no longer needed a scooter to move about. Rudy was able to return to his medical practice as an emergency room physician. To this day, he believes that his erroneous MS diagnosis would have condemned him to a shortened, inferior quality of life. He is incredibly happy that using the frequencies of his voice as a guide, the computer analysis was able to reveal the definitive mathematical cause for his lack of wellness.

Rudy's case history is an example of how each person's Signature Sound is influenced by his or her genetic make-up and the environment in which he or she lives. It reflects an individual's physical, mental/emotional, and spiritual state, and includes the sound that is produced otoacoustically by the ears. As Rachel Yehuda, MD, Professor of Psychiatry and Neuroscience, and Director of the Traumatic Stress Studies Division at the Icahn School of Medicine at Mount Sinai, has stated, "Speech has a unique signature that could also be captured with other markers, such as blood biomarkers, identifying a 'unique' fingerprint."

Over the last few decades, data collection by my Institute of BioAcoustic Biology has successfully provided the proof that persons who experience parallel issues (traumas, diseases, genetic issues, immuno-suppression, psychological stresses, toxins, pathogens, etc) have similar, if not identical, anomalous vocal mathematical patterns. They are frequency relationships that could be considered akin to a "sour" note in a song.

Human BioAcoustics is based on the theory that the brain communicates using the language of Frequency Equivalents™ which are numeric representations of people, places, or things. Studies show that the Vocal Profile protocol I developed provides the opportunity to reveal individual health-related numeric templates, which have the potential to promote and extend life. Over decades, hundreds of numeric patterns of the voice have been decoded by myself and my dedicated co-workers.

From birth to death, we use sounds to express our needs and emotions, but there are additional layers of information hidden within the words. In modern times, we possess only limited conscious awareness of this information for ourselves or as a means to interpret the intentions of others. Vocal Profiling software has been developed that can use the components of the voice to create a matrix of information about anyone, from fundamental DNA, to the hidden intentions of those who claim to speak for us.

Our brain is a central processing unit of our body that initiates and circulates frequencies throughout our vast neural networks; providing directives and power to keep our bodies in exacting homeostasis (healthy balance). This indicates that even unspoken thought can become our guiding force in keeping us healthy and emotionally well-balanced. (And also potentially controlled through electronic means.) We are on the precipice of learning to use the individual sounds exhibited by the body as intrinsic, individual healing directives.

For centuries, curious minds have attempted to compare sounds, light, emotions, and disease states with the health and maladies of the human condition. Finding your own voice takes on new meaning if you begin to consider the possibility that the sounds of your voice may be a holographic representation of all that you are.

From birth to death, we use sounds to express our needs and emotions but there are additional layers of information hidden within our words. As humans evolved, language became levels of intricate harmony nestled within structures of great elegance that carried meaning and allowed understanding of ourselves and others. Everything that happens to the body reaches the brain as bio-frequencies that are then sorted, routed, and assigned an interpretation

And there actually is an ear focus involved in this process, as well.

If you listen to me talk, then listen to something in another room, or the outside traffic, then listen to me again, you can hear or feel your ear focus change. We're all very much aware of how our eye focus changes when looking at something close, and then far away, but most people do not realize that a similar change of focus occurs in the ear. When you begin to consciously change that focus of your ear, you'll start hearing a very high pitch sound, which I believe is your Signature Sound—the frequency representation of all that you are. Everything that's ever happened to you is manifested in that sound.

What we have found through voice spectral analysis is that when a person is not in an optimum state of health, both physiologically and psychologically, his or her voice will have missing notes or tones that are part of one's Signature Sound. Indicators of physical and/or mental/emotional distress can then be categorized from these notes, and when the sound frequencies that correspond to them are provided, the ability to self-heal is significantly enhanced.

In other words, in a healthy state, a Signature Sound would be vibrant and contain the full spectrum of notes that comprise it, but in a state of illness something in the frequency would be lacking or off. Or too high, or too choppy. We've run tests on this.

During the Human BioAcoustics' process, when you present someone with their Signature Sound, it will synchronize their heart and brain. Your heart and your brain will synchronize to the beat frequency of it. I think the frequency is actually coming from your brain, but the rhythm of the sound is actually coming from your heart. When you listen to your own sound, it brings harmony and balance to the different systems of the body and is very relaxing. When we do the computer analysis, it gives us everything that makes up the Signature Sound. Almost like a chord.

The Power of the Voice to Heal

It was a life emergency that forced me to reveal the full potential of the abilities I was born with to the world.

My sacred story eludes me because my unusual talent was present before my memory begins. And I still don't know how my ability to make history by creating the future will evolve.

During the course of my life, no one acknowledged that I was different or that I had talents beyond normal human abilities. Perhaps being raised in the foothills of Appalachia may have been the impetus for my unique hearing and vocal abilities. My adoptive parents didn't understand how I knew what the animals needed or wanted. Nor did they understand why headaches dissipated when I hummed or sang peculiar notes, or knew where the water was in any forest, when a crop was willing to be harvested, or how I was able to explain what people weren't saying, all because of what I could hear that others could not. All of that was far beyond my own understanding, at the time. I didn't know I was unique. And even if I did know, who would I tell? Growing up, visitors were few and far between.

To my knowledge, my unusual abilities were not discussed even with family. My caretakers may have been concerned that I would be intimidating to some people so they kept me away from others, cautioning me about talking to anyone, and even delaying my entrance into school.

Though my abilities have subsequently been substantiated in many university and military labs, at first I didn't understand that I hear beyond the normal human range or how my voice creates pure tone, something that supposedly is impossible for a human voice.

It is supposedly a fact that a person can only vocally reproduce what they hear, and essentially I was only hearing the sounds of nature. In my early years, we had no electricity, no running water, and no radio.

The sounds I hear turned out to be the morphogenic resonance of plants and described as a Signature Sound in ancient healing literature, and as otoacoustic emissions by modern science.

Although I was hoping that my children would inherit my unique talents, that doesn't seem to be the case. So I set about using computer advancements to help duplicate what I was hearing and am able to vocally reproduce.

I didn't want what I was capable of doing to die with me. The information had served me well even though I often treated my talent with indifference using it when I needed it and hiding it from others most of the time.

The time came when I was forced to display my talent for an audience. My 16-year-old daughter had slipped off a 12 foot-high rope as she swung in the air like Tarzan. She fell into a few inches of water. When I got to her from across the isolated, but crowded swimming hole, her lower leg was hanging off to one side. I knew instantly that I was going to either watch her bleed to death or reveal what I could do in public.

I twisted her leg back together, wrapped it tightly in a tee-shirt, had people help me bring her to the river bank, and starting making sounds. I don't know if people stood back in awe or fear. I already knew that if I just let go and allowed the energy to flow through me that the right sounds would somehow flow through my vocal cords. The sounds I produced saved my daughter's life.

The doctors can't explain why she didn't bleed to death because we were 45 minutes away from help, and her leg was hanging on by a large artery that had also been damaged. The hospital ordeal lasted over a month, with four operations plus months of recuperation, but her leg is now intact and serves her well, considering the extent of the damages.

Because of that experience, I knew that the talent that I had been treating frivolously deserved to be respected, even revered. As a result, I committed myself to learning how this could be real, and how it could help others. I vowed to discover how it happened, why it happened, and how it worked. I grieved that I could not explain the science behind what had happened. If I could save one parent from having to watch their child die, I would dedicate my life to discovering how sound could influence the energy body and dictate its reactions to trauma, stress, and disease.

The energy body is real. Taming and understanding it will reveal how frequency is an ancient mystery being revealed as we attempt to understand the potential of math as medicine: the medicine of the future.

I can hear and duplicate the sounds and frequencies that people need to balance and become well. My mission today is to provide tools and solutions to the public in the hopes of making a difference, and, perhaps selfishly, I hope that my time on the planet will leave it a better place.

Mysteries of the Voice

A few years ago, I was unceremoniously dumped as a speaker at an international sound healing conference. The justification offered was that I had no musical talent and therefore would not be an informative nor entertaining speaker. It is likely that I have one of the most unusual "musical" talents on the planet and that my "no talent" abilities have the potential to change human history.

I can actively hear tones and music emanating from people and I can duplicate the tones I hear as pure tones, even though this is something considered impossible for the human voice to reproduce.

I hear these sounds not from people's voices but from their ears. Providing people their own Signature Sounds via ambient or mechanical means seems to provide an innate, individual restorative agenda for each person. This unusual talent has led to the uncovering of information about human physiology that may make our future survival more feasible. It may seem like the stuff of Star Trek medicine, but it is available now.

Even though I was jolted by being disinvited from the conference, I refused to be put off. From my own past experiences, I knew that the tones I heard and sang to my daughter had saved her life, helped relieve pain, assisted in reconstituting human tissue, restored nerve function, influenced emotions, and helped people recover from disease, and, as in the case of Rudy above, walk again. These events show that there is so much more to these Signature Sounds than people realize.

When examined using an oscilloscope, the vibrations of the sounds I sing create pictures. My research has shown that individual tones can be diagnostically supportive, have long-term health implications, and show that frequency can create form. But more importantly, these innate mechanisms of sound frequencies need to be understood in order to elevate our knowledge of the planet and our existence.

The adage that our voice and thoughts can create reality is true.

Is my ability to hear Signature Sounds a useful talent?

I had never heard of anyone else hearing music coming from a person's ears.

Is this an ancient talent that humans lost or is it a future talent that is just now being embraced?

Sylvia Franke, author of *The Tree of Life and the Holy Grail*, claims that I am a "modern keeper of the Holy Grail information", so we can suppose that this is an ancient, forgotten talent being brought back into fruition.

Research conduction at Johns Hopkins University has confirmed that the ear emits a sound called an otoacoustic emission. My ears have been tested in university and military labs, confirming that I'm hearing the otoacoustic emissions that are consistently being emitted by, not just people, but by living systems. Not only can I hear the sounds, but I can also duplicate the sounds accurately to two decimal points as pure sine waves.

I can also hear the sounds of a room's dimension and from the sound predict the dimensions of the room, combining sound and geometry. This method emulates the mathematical relationship of musical notes, and opens the idea that room dimensions could create sounds in a room that is below normal hearing but useful for healing.

With training, people can hear their own otoacoustic emissions. Would being able to hear and interpret your own sounds to facilitate complete wellness be useful?

From the studies that have attempted to interpret individual otoacoustic emissions in support of optimal health, it has been determined that the sounds from the ears are mimicked by the voice and that, from measurements of its frequencies, frequency-based solutions can be created and quantified. Does this mean that frequency-based tones could be used for healing?

The answer to that questions is most definitely yes. That fact has been proven and validated numerous times by myself and those I have trained in Human BioAcoustics as we employ Vocal Profiling and use sound frequencies to help people reverse a wide range of health conditions.

Dorinne Davis, MA, author of *Sound Bodies Through Sound Therapy*, helps children regain speech. She is involved with the Alfred Tomatis method of evaluating otoacoustic emissions to assist in regaining brain function and language. Her studies have proven that 100 percent of the time, the voice emulates the tones being emitted by the ear.

Similarly, the science of Cymatics postulates, and can prove, that frequency vibrations can animate small particles into geometric shapes. My ears can "hear" the shape of a room and, based on its dimensions, can identify its architecture. If I "sing" the exact harmonics of a space, an echo is created.

Many ancient architectural enclosures are considered to be healing. How much did the ancients who built them know about that we just do not remember?

The knowledge that the tones I created, as musical notes, could make people physically weak or strong set me on a quest that led to Susan Alexjander, who set human DNA to musical notes (see her Sequencia album), and James Gimzewski, a UCLA professor who has proven that living cells create sound. Alexjander's group created haunting music based on the frequencies of DNA, and Gimzewski stated that if we could figure out the cellular sounds of humans it would change the face of medicine, allowing us to "fix" ourselves using different frequency formats. I believe the ancients knew this because humans throughout recorded history used frequency as music to heal and soothe.

If You Can Moan, You Can Tone

From the first wail at birth to the funeral lament, sound and rhythm are a part of our lives. In between these two moments, we use a variety of notes, pitch and intonation to express ourselves. Some of these vocalizations are learned; others are quite natural and spontaneous.

All manner of systems have been devised to organize the various sounds we produce. Language and musical composition are probably the two most well-known. Techniques such as toning, praying, chanting, and primal screaming are just a few of the methods that have been used in our attempts to gain dominion over our physical and emotional selves. But it is the natural tones that seem to be the most useful. These sounds are associated with the most fundamental aspects of our lives, and we didn't have to learn them. They represent an untapped means of gaining dominion over our physical and emotional selves. Granted, however, they are the ones that we often don't use, at least not in public.

The natural grunts, groans and sighs are the sounds used when we find ourselves in our most vulnerable states—when we are ill, afraid, grieving, angry, or making love—yet we often don't use them, at least not in public. These sounds are associated with the most fundamental aspects of our lives. We didn't have to learn to moan or weep. It is not required that someone teach us to groan or laugh. With few exceptions, the ability to produce such sounds comes as standard equipment in humans, and first gain expression right after we are born.

One type of vocal expression that has particular significance when it comes to healing is what is known as toning, which, along with chanting, has been a part of religious, spiritual, and healing traditions since time immemorial.

Almost anyone can tone. Try it now. Make a sound, any sound, it doesn't matter which kind. Make the sound originate from your throat, your nose, from deep in your gut. Now close your mouth and continue making a sound.

Do you feel the sound moving and vibrating through your nose?

Experiment with this. Run a scale from the lowest to the highest note you can make.

Do you like one sound better than the other?

Does one tone make you vibrate more than the others?

The sounds that cause you to vibrate are the most helpful. Vibrating tones in your sinus cavity or throat have been known to reduce the pain of a headache and decrease sinus, ear, or throat infections.

Puff out your cheeks and blow a sound through your, barely touching, front teeth. See if you can find a note that will make your teeth or inner ear vibrate. Congratulations, you just learned to how to tone your own Signature Sound!

Even professional speech therapists are now admitting that the sound of your voice has a lot to do with your energy and health. Just open your mouth and make a sound; a noise. It doesn't have to make sense, even to you. It doesn't need to be pleasing to anyone but you. Although some people may want you to believe that toning must be done in a special form or fashion, don't believe it. No one is better at moaning (or toning) for you than you are.

Working With A Person's Signature Sound

The Vocal Profiling system I developed enables anyone trained in the practice of Human BioAcoustics to quickly come to know everything that makes up a person's Signature Sound, and to then be able to present it back to them in a way that creates a state of harmony.

There are actually two frequency or sound formulas that are required. One is a formula based on the molecular weight of the compound or body part that we are targeting, and the other is a formula based on a frequency that will engage the energy of the compound or body part.

As an analogy to this, consider a car. When you start the engine, the car is ready to go, but in order to put it into action, you have to put it into gear and step on the gas. This is similar to how we use these two sound frequencies with the people we see.

The first frequency alerts the compound or body part that we're about to engage its energy, and the second one actually does engage the energy, allowing us to control how much of that energy is expended. For instance, what we have found during a pilot study is that, if someone requires a particular compound, such as a nutrient, we can call that up and engage its sound frequency and then present that sound frequency to the person, and the body will react just as if the person had taken the nutrient orally. Moreover, instead of the body having to digest the nutrient itself before it can be utilized, when we introduce the nutrient's corresponding sound frequency, the reaction and its positive effects will be immediate. And by being able to shut the frequency off, we can avoid any side-effects the compound might otherwise cause. We would like to do more work to explore this potential.

Toning and Discovering Your Signature Sound

I created the following exercises as a means of helping people to work with sound to enhance vitality, and for discovering your own Signature Sound.

To discover your Signature Sound, first try this exercise: Listen for a few seconds to a sound that is very near to you. Now change your focus and listen to a sound that is several feet away, or in another room. Now listen close again. Now far.

As you keep changing your focus between the near and far sounds, notice if you can feel your ears changing their focus as well. With practice, you will be able to. Eventually, you will begin to hear a high pitched ring in your ear, one that you could not possibly match vocally. It is present in your ear and you can hear it if you know how to listen.

If you haven't heard such a ring, maybe you haven't trained your ear to focus. This is your own personal sound, your own Soul Note or Signature Sound. This is your own intrinsic frequency that animates you and keeps you alive and manifests as your Energy Body. It is exactly right for you, every minute of every day, and listening to it will feed you the tones you need. every moment of every day.

Another way to listen to your Signature Sound is to lay down and place a pillow over each ear, then listen as you practice changing your hearing focus. If you have difficulty hearing your sound this way, try making a very low note and then slowly slide up and down the scale as you listen for your ears to rings.

You can also practice this while cupping your hands over your ears. Once your ears start to ring, stop making any sound and listen to the tones inside your ears. Actively listening to these patterns will take you into a theta brain wave state which, according to researcher Dr. Robert Becker, is the level of the body's healing range.

Conclusion

My work has shown that we can each have dominion over our frequencies by individual mind management, or a simple remote control that is completely programmable. In the near future, I believe that bio-frequencies, as an indicator of health, will become as common as taking your temperature or blood pressure, when you visit your health care provider. MIT, the Mayo Clinic, and several universities, are already working with these principles, and AT&T has declared that "bioacoustics is the medicine of the future."

This ancient idea of Signature Sounds combined with modern techniques of Vocal Profiling can enable the body to identify and prescribe for itself using the algorithms of vocalized frequencies to accurately quantify, organize, and extrapolate biometric information. Through entrainment of the frequency grids of the brain, the body can be programmed to support its own optimal form and function.

CHAPTER 3

THE BODY AS A MATHEMATICAL SOUND MATRIX—USING THE UNIVERSAL LAWS OF HARMONICS TO HEAL

Both science and religion agree that everything is frequency and that frequency is everything. Science shares this thought by stating that the most common denominator of all structure, the atom, is energy, a form of frequency. In the Bible, which is considered the Word of God, it is stated, "In the beginning was the Word, and the Word was with God, and the Word was God" (John 1:1). Since sound is also frequency, God joins science in the observation that at its foundation, frequency is the basis of our universe.

Frequency is emotion.

Frequency is muscle strength and weakness.

Frequency is electrical impulses.

Frequency is magnetic potential.

Frequency is neuromuscular currents.

Frequency is aroma. Frequency is sound.

Frequency is light.

Frequency is vibration.

Frequency, in short, is everything!

In this chapter, I will explain how frequency and mathematics tie together and how our physical bodies can be considered as mathematical sound matrices. Let's begin by discussing sound itself.

What Is Sound?

Professor David Q. Naiman of the Department of Applied Mathematics and Statistics at John Hopkins University, defines sound as "the rapid cycling between compression and rarefaction of air". He further explains, "The way that sounds move through the air can be thought of as analogous to the way vibrations move along a slinky. The metal parts of the slinky don't move from one end to the other. What does move along the slinky as it vibrates, is the regions where the spring is compressed or stretched out. The same thing happens when air is compressed for an instant. The air molecules themselves do not move very far, but wave of high density air moves at the speed of sound, roughly 770 miles per hour. To represent such cyclic behavior mathematically, think of the air pressure at a listener's location as a function of time described by a sine wave or sinusoid... one can use such signals as basic building blocks for some truly interesting forms of sound. So it is essential to understand these key building blocks and how they combine to form complex sounds.

"A sinusoid can be thought of in geometrical terms as follows. Imagine a point moving counter-clockwise around the unit circle at a constant speed...The speed at which the point rotates about the origin can be measured in terms of the number of complete cycles made per second. This quantity is referred to as the sinusoid's frequency... When sound waves are combined, the results can be quite complicated, yet, our ears are able to disentangle some sound components and hear them as separate units." (Naiman DQ. *Mathematics of Music.* www.ams.jhu.edu/dan-mathofmusic/sound-waves)

In an article entitled *The Mathematics Behind Sound*, Mickey Hart, the famed musician and percussionist and former band member of The Grateful Dead, stated, "Scientifically speaking, sound is nothing more than the vibratory movement of air molecules. But the variations in how such vibrations occur are nearly limitless, creating every sound imaginable, and all the world's musical traditions.

"Determining and calculating these variables allow someone to understand the mathematics behind sound. Many of the variables which contribute to a sound's particular quality are measurable thanks to the work of scientists and mathematicians who have created systems that allow us to calculate sound in various ways. These variables include:

"Amplitude measures the volume of a sound. In musical terms, it is often known as dynamics. Amplitude is calculated in decibels, a logarithmic scale, and measured over time with a level meter.

"Envelope defines how the amplitude of a sound changes over time. In musical terms, envelope is often described as articulation. It is measured in decibels in time (usually milliseconds), and is often visually represented and analyzed as a waveform.

"Frequency defines how high or low a sound is. It is called pitch in musical terminology, and is measured in hertz. The frequency of a sound can be calculated by dividing the rate of the compressions and rarefactions by the length of a sound wave. An oscilloscope is an electronic device that is often used to measure and visualize a sound's frequency.

"Spectrum represents how many different frequencies a sound produces. Most of the instruments and objects that create sound vibrate in multiple ways, creating not a single frequency, but a spectrum of frequencies. The various frequencies a sound produces can be measured in decibels, creating a spectrogram of the sound. A spectrometer is often used to measure the frequency spectrum of a sound over time.

Comprehending and being able to calculate the mathematics behind sound—including amplitude, envelope, frequency, and spectrum—not only leads to a deeper understanding into the physical nature of sound, but is also essential knowledge for musicians and audio engineers who seek to express themselves through sound."
(Source: *https://teachrocklessonpdf.s3.amazonaws.com/Music+and+Math/The+ Mathematics+Behind+Sound_Printable+Lesson_v3.pdf*)

The famed jazz pianist and composer Thelonious Monk also recognized the relationship between music and math when he stated, "All musicians are subconsciously mathematicians."

To which I would add that comprehending and being able to calculate the mathematics behind sound is also essential knowledge that I discovered and used to pioneer Human BioAcoustics for the purposes of sound healing. The mathematics of frequency is also how and why the Vocal Profiling system I developed is able to mathematically detect and analyze everything that a person's voice reveals about her or his overall state of health and their body's nutritional status.

The Music of the Spheres

As I noted above, frequency is the basis of our universe. I mean that literally, and so does the scientific community, whose research has proven that everything within the universe is in a state of perpetual vibration.

The ancients, including Pythagoras of Samos, the 6th century BC sage Greek philosopher and mathematician, recognized this fact long ago. Pythagoras taught that the proportions in the movements of the Sun, Moon and planets was due to what became known as the "music, or harmony, of the spheres". In Pythagoras's view, the Sun, Moon, and planets all produced their own unique tone or hum during their orbital revolutions. Pythagoras also taught that mathematical relationships expressed specific tones or frequencies of energy that are found in numbers, shapes, and visual angles, as well as in all sounds. He was also the first person to discover that the pitch of a musical note is an inverse proportion to the length of the string of the instrument that produces it.

Commenting on Pythagoras's teachings, Aristotle wrote, "Some thinkers suppose that the motion of bodies of that size must produce a noise, since on our earth the motion of bodies far inferior in size and in speed of movement has that effect. Also, when the sun and the moon, they say, and all the stars, so great in number and in size, are moving with so rapid a motion, how should they not produce a sound immensely great?

Starting from this argument and from the observation that their speeds, as measured by their distances, are in the same ratios as musical concordances, they assert that the sound given forth by the circular movement of the stars is a harmony. Since, however, it appears unaccountable that we should not hear this music, they explain this by saying that the sound is in our ears from the very moment of birth and is thus indistinguishable from its contrary silence, since sound and silence are discriminated by mutual contrast. What happens to men, then, is just what happens to coppersmiths, who are so accustomed to the noise of the smithy that it makes no difference to them." (*Aristotle. "Book 2, Part 9". On the Heavens.*)

However, it must be said that Aristotle rejected the idea of the music of the spheres because it did not fit with his own model of the cosmos. Science, however, has since proven that Pythagoras was right. NASA, for example, recorded all planet sounds from space in the form of electromagnetic vibration and converted into the audible range of human ear: 20-20,000 Hz.

As Elizabeth Landau, of NASA's Exoplanet Exploration Program, explains, "We can't hear it with our ears, but the stars in the sky are performing a concert, one that never stops. The biggest stars make the lowest, deepest sounds, like tubas and double basses. Small stars have high-pitched voices, like celestial flutes. These virtuosos don't just play one 'note' at a time, either—our own Sun has thousands of different sound waves bouncing around inside it at any given moment.

"Understanding these stellar harmonies represents a revolution in astronomy. By 'listening' for stellar sound waves with telescopes, scientists can figure out what stars are made of, how old they are, how big they are and how they contribute to the evolution of our Milky Way galaxy as a whole. The technique is called asteroseismology. Just as earthquakes (or Earth's seismic waves) tell us about the inside of Earth, stellar waves—resulting in vibrations or 'star quakes'—reveal the secret inner workings of stars."

This concept of music of the spheres was for centuries accepted by and carried down to other philosophers and scientists, including the renowned 16th-century astronomer Johannes Kepler, who further developed this concept. NASA's Kepler space telescope, named after him, played a key role in the field of asteroseismology, "delivering observations of waves in tens of thousands of stars after its 2009 launch," according to Landau.

Math As Medicine

As I pointed out above, frequency is the basis of our universe. We measure it, study it, quantify it, and use it to understand ourselves, our environment, our biochemistry, and our behaviors. But what if there were more to our origins? What if frequency (the measurement of vibration and frequency), the basis of everything, is more than synthetic equations?

What if math is organic?

If so, could we be considered math-based life forms?

Consider the brain as the central processing unit of our bodies. Frequency-based signals are generated and have been determined to be a communication pathway traveling along our neural networks that self-monitor and keep our bodies in homeostasis (the self-regulating process by which humans and all other living organisms maintain a stable internal environment despite ongoing changes in external conditions).

We know that frequency can be represented in terms of mathematical equations. Does this fact indicate that math could be a form of healing? If math can be proven to be a form of healing, does this indicate that math may be organic and that our human forms that our Creator created came about through the use of a Divine type of mathematics?

My research indicates that this may be the case, and that math can be used as medicine. I believe that at our core we are very sophisticated math-based beings, and that we can be "managed" through our individual frequency/energy-based Signature Sounds. My work at the Institute of BioAcoustic Biology & Sound Health has shown that we can each have dominion over those frequencies by individual mind management or by using specific sound frequencies and the tone boxes that I've developed that are completely programmable.

It was Pythagoras who observed that if one of two strings of the same length and which have the same degree of tension, is then divided in half, that the half string, when played, creates a harmonic exactly one octave higher than the longer string. As Pythagoras continued to divide the string into ratios of 1:2, 1:3, 1-:4, etc., he was able to observe the principles of sound that we called harmonics that still govern much of the music theory in use today. The discovery of the mathematical relationships underlying the science of sound clearly demonstrated that harmonics were not an abstract concept but adhered to strict and predictable mathematical principles. These very same principles govern much of our music experience today. Pythagoras and his followers proposed that the body be subject to the same harmonic laws that govern music.

The modern day principles of Human BioAcoustics have successfully combined these two ideas. What is emerging is a new science that recognizes the body's structure and function as a mathematical harmonic matrix. Repeatable studies have shown that human biology and interactions conform to a prescribed set of Body Harmonics.

Here is an example of what I mean:

The suggestion that the number 8 is the opposite of the number 11 (more specifically, 11.3136) is a foreign notion to most people. No such model is taught in school but the reality is that our body knows this concept to be true and responds to numbers and frequencies in its attempt to conduct the normal homeostatic processes of the body.

Actually, mathematical opposites are easily understood when one considers other forms of opposites recognized by both Science and the Arts. Each color has an opposite known as a pigment or light complement. Red and green are complementary colors by pigment. Noise cancelling head sets are an example of pigment complements working together. But red and turquoise are light complements. The differences are in pigment and light refraction. And each color can be represented by a frequency.

The frequencies, which represent complementary colors, could be considered Frequency Complements™.

Just as green and red are opposite or complementary colors, there are green frequencies (in the frequency range of 11) and red frequencies (in the frequency range of 8). Using this concept, an overabundance of the frequency of 11 can be equalized by using the frequency of 8 and vice-versa. By using 8 (or any frequency we choose as a base) we can begin to construct formulas that the body uses innately to provide balance and healing. This is apparent in the research I've conducted by Sound Health Inc., an educational research institute located in USA, in southeastern Ohio. Over many years of developmental research and two decades of studies, using data from vocal analysis has shown that every muscle, every tissue and organ, every compound, every process and structure of the body has a Frequency Equivalent™ that can be mathematically calculated. This calculation is the basis of Human BioAcoustics, which indicates that the body's ability to heal itself originates as an interaction, whether bio-chemical and/or structural, that is a predictable mathematical response.

For example, we all know that calcium and magnesium are used together in the body. When you combine the Frequency Equivalents™ of calcium and magnesium, the Frequency Equivalent™ of phosphorus is the result. Phosphorus is one of the compounds that is required for calcium and magnesium to be able to act together synergistically.

As another example, the Frequency Equivalent™ of choline used together with its complement creates the Frequency Equivalent™ of ace-tylcholine. This imitates the reactions of the body that science has already discovered: that choline is used to create acetylcholine.

Human biology and the Frequency Equivalents™ of the mathematical matrix of the body emulate each other. One of the frequencies that have been shown to be able to strengthen the thumb, for instance, is the note of C. By presenting the specific note within the note of C that is required, it can be shown that the thumb muscles become stronger. Giving the Frequency Complement™ of the same muscle will cause the muscle to weaken. Since the Frequency Equivalent™ of the thumb muscle happens to correspond to the Frequency Equivalent™ of zinc, the body will also accept the compound of zinc as a support for that muscle. Our physical bodies are apparently built on, and correspond to, a blueprint created by thousands of these combinations. Each organ, muscle, nutrient or bio-chemical has a Frequency Equivalent™ that is interrelated via the body's central processing unit, the brain and nervous system. A vocal print can show that a combination of notes and the corresponding frequencies can be used to create the coherent mathematically patterns that are required by our bodies. When these patterns become dissonant, *dis-ease* is the result. And when these patterns harmonize, they support health and well-being.

How simple then to monitor and maintain our own health through a daily review of our vocal prints. This is something you can easily learn how to do, as will be explained later in this book.

In addition to viewing the body as a mathematical matrix, Human BioAcoustics considers the idea that frequencies can be used to predict states of disease and stress before they become obvious on a physical level. Protocols have been developed by me to identify the frequency relationships for cancer, heart disease, arthritis, and sports injuries for example. And I am continuing to develop additional protocols to identify other conditions.

The study of numerous vocal prints permits researchers to recognize obvious frequency markers for various state of illness. Some frequencies are apparently more important to our states of health than others. The frequency of 16.00, as an example, is a very important internal frequency since it can help release oxygen and calcium into the cells. In his book, *Cross Currents*, Robert Becker, MD, stated that calcium, which is released by the frequency of 16.00 cycles per second, is an important nutrient in the healing process of the body. The most compelling information concern-ing 16.00 cycles per second of frequency may change medicine and the way we treat disease. This is the concept of harmonics.

The number 16 itself proves to be an important number in this pro-cess of harmonics. Starting with a fundamental frequency of a note, the mathematically determined series of notes that have been identified as the harmonics of each note are listed below. Notice that each list has 16 steps beyond the fundamental. The last note is exactly one octave higher than the first, just as in the principle of octaves, wherein each octave is exactly double the previous octave.

HARMONIC SERIES OF NOTES

```
C C# D D# E F F# G G# A A# B
G G# A A# B C C# D D# E F F#
C C# D D# E F F# G G# A A# B
E F F# G G# A A# B C C# D D#
G G# A A# B C C# D D# E F F#
A# B C C# D D# E F F# G G# A
C C# D D# E F F# G G# A A# B
D D# E F F# G G# A A# B C C#
E F F# G G# A A# B C C# D D#
F# G G# A A# B C C# D D# E F
G G# A A# B C C# D D# E F F#
G# A A# B C C# D D# E F F# G
A# B C C# D D# E F F# G G# A
B C C# D D# E F F# G G# A A#
C C# D D# E F F# G G# A A# B
```

(Note: Unless the midpoint of a note range is used, the frequency note correlates may not always fall within the prescribed label for the note. This is due to the uneven ratios of the scale from which this particular table was derived.)

When played in a series or together, mathematical harmonics are not esthetically pleasing to most people. Our senses tell us that music created by ratios, such as the even-tempered scale, are much more pleasing to the ear. Thus, mathematical harmonics have not been used in musical composition. These precise harmonics, however, used in combination with the Frequency Equivalents™ discovered through Human BioAcoustic research, form an intricate harmonic synergy that maintains what I call the SonoStatis that is essential for optimal health. Our body functions as a compilation of frequencies and frequency relationships. The brain functions through the use of brain waves, which are measurable as frequency. The heart also emits frequency to keep the heart beating in rhythm. Nerve transmission is accomplished through the use of frequency pathways, as well.

Organs, nerves, tissue and bone, are themselves made up of substances, which are at their base, energy that is measurable in cycles per second. The body is alive, literally, with frequencies that interact in cooperative resonance and harmony.

The following example illustrates how the combination of fundamental harmonics combined with the concept of the Frequency Equivalent™ of Human BioAcoustics would work. Use any number; 26 for example. Divide that number 26 by 2 until the result is a number between 1 and 2, in this case 1.625. This is called the fundamental. Start with the first multiple in the hearing range of your original number, in this case, 26, and add 1.625 to that number 16 times.

HARMONIC FUNDAMENTAL LISTING FOR THE NUMBER 26:

26.
27.625
29.25
30.875
32.5
34.125
35.75
37.375
39.00
40.625
42.25
43.875

45.5

47.125

48.75

50.375

52.

As you can see, the 16th multiple creates a double of the original number, a harmonic that is one octave above. More importantly, the listing of numbers that are created contains the Frequency Equivalents™ of the compounds and structures that are involved in the body's use of the original number, 26.

This is one set of frequencies that are used. The others are all notes in a scale.

All of the Frequency Equivalents™ that correspond to the use of nutrients and biochemicals that relate to this particular harmonic set can now be used to evaluate the efficacy of the interactions involved. The list names all of the compounds, interactions, muscles, tendons, nerves, ligaments, etc. which are involved in the transmission and use of the information contained in that particular harmonic set.

This mathematical matrix maps the crossroads of alchemy and cooperation between the different systems of the body. If a mineral, fatty acid, amino acid, biochemical or enzyme, for example, have similar frequencies, they may all participate as nearly interchangeable components performing the same work.

Consider sulfur and palmitic acid, for example, which are similar Frequency Equivalents™. They can substitute for each other in the fight against invading pathogens. Other compounds that are found within the same harmonic set react in a similar fashion. The body is adept at compensating, substituting, and transmuting frequencies. If an enzyme isn't available to help counter invading pathogens, fatty acids and minerals can be substituted. In the same way, Frequency Equivalents™ harmonic sets can be used to establish substitutes using mathematical matrix relationships. This means that if we construct a harmonic set for the Frequency Equivalents of Vitamin C, we can use this listing to observe every other compound that interacts with Vitamin C and, in addition, see the structural aspects most affected by Vitamin C.

During clinic trials, we have been able to present a frequency to a subject and watch the Frequency Equivalents of compounds that are influenced by them by monitoring the subject's vocal print. In many instances, the interactions were previously unknown. For example, in a study that was conducted to determine the originating factors of knee problem in tennis players, it was found that the knee was not the actual root cause. The base problem turned out to be a muscle in the foot. Human BioAcoustic research indicates that standardized harmonic sets could be used to predict, depict, and monitor the chemical and behavioral interactions and relationships of all living systems.

When all of the Frequency Equivalents of compounds and physiology are known, every aspect of any one frequency can be studied. We will comprehend and understand frequency relationships and how they all relate to each other. Then we will be able to develop an elemental frequency grid similar to the elemental table of compounds. We have created software that shows the deep inner relationships of any given frequency.

Every compound has a Frequency Equivalent. Presenting a Frequency Equivalent in analog form to the body allows the body to recognize the presence of that compound. When an additional frequency, based on a mathematical formula of the Frequency Equivalent is presented, the substance becomes functional, meaning it is able to be used by the body. A Frequency Equivalent that allows this awareness by the brain is called a Brain Wave Multiple (BWM). In disease, the body may not have the necessary brain wave multiples to identify or stimulate a compound or muscle. A Frequency Equivalent can provide the brain wave multiples that act to stimulate the detection and function of a compound or structure.

(Note: It is imperative that brain wave multiples be presented in an analog, not digital, form. According to Robert O. Becker and many others, the body's input mechanisms are analog and respond most efficiently to analog sounds.)

To see this technique in action is quite extraordinary. The following case history from Human BioAcoustic clinical files show the potential of this work. (Many more case histories are presented in the next chapter.)

A female jogger was referred to the Human BioAcoustic clinic because one of her legs was two inches shorter than the other due to an accident. An operation was scheduled to attempt to elongate the bone. We were able to discover by evaluating her vocal print that a thigh muscle was very restrained. We relaxed the muscle using low frequency analog sound frequencies.

Within a few minutes of exercise both of her legs were the same length and they have continued, with exercise, to remain normalized.

What could this technique provide as predictive medicine?

Could heart attacks be predicted?

Could an exact time of birth be more closely determined by monitoring the hormone levels of the expectant mother?

Could we become a planet of healthy people because we could predict trends and move to prevent disease before its symptoms become evident?

Could this technology allow us to become more aware of our environment?

We as a society have created many of our own disease issues by our innovations. For instance, the frequency created by fluorescent lights is a frequency that is also associated with prostate cancer.

A recent issue of the *Advance Journal for Audiologists* reported that vocal patterns are often an indicator of states of health. Listening to digital sounds and the carrier wave hidden within them can actually create interference in your vocal patterns. Human BioAcoustics is a new, developing science. Not all of the answers are obvious but there is enough known information to show the establishment of definitive patterns for states of disease. Dr. Andy Weil, Dr. Robert O. Becker, Dr. William Tillis, Dr. Alfred Tomatis and Dr. Richard Gerber, among other distinguished medical practitioners, all agree that frequency and rhythm, as various forms of energy, can be important aspects of knowing and healing the body.

The Body and Octaves

The human body utilizes several levels, or octaves, that enable it to communicate with itself, and also enable us to communicate with other. These octaves, provided in specific combinations, also allow the body's different systems to communicate and cooperate with each other.

These octave levels are as follows:

01 – 02 cycles per second (CPS): biomagnetic.
02 – 04 CPS: bioelectric.
04 – 08 CPS: biochemical.
08 – 16 CPS: emotional.
16 – 32 CPS: structural/muscular.
32 – 64 CPS: neuro-physical.
64 – 128 CPS: connective tissue.

The vocal print diagnostic methodology I developed has the ability to determine the root cause of emotional distress and physical disease by showing the frequencies of each octave. If a frequency in a certain octave is high it means that there is too much energy in that octave and for that frequency. For a muscle, this would mean that the muscle is too tight. For a compound, it indicates overabundance or excess. Conversely. if there is not enough energy in the octave frequency, this is an indication of a deficiency. Health, both physical and mental/emotional, occurs when there is neither an overabundance or deficiency, a state of balance. This concept is well-known by practitioners of traditional Chinese medicine (TCM) in which optimal health is regarded as a balance of *yin* and *yang* energies in the body's meridian pathways and organ systems.

As we study the human voice, we find that these octave frequencies are an intrinsic part of the formula that must be provided for health to occur and be maintained. But just as important as the frequencies themselves are the rhythm format that must be used.

The Mathematical Harmonic Matrix

The modern day principles of Human BioAcoustics is leading to an emerging new science that perceives the body's structure and function as a mathematical harmonic matrix. Repeatable studies have shown that human biology and interactions conform to a prescribed set of Body Harmonics. The concept of harmonics state that every note has a set of corresponding notes or frequencies that are created when the original note is created. While Pythagoras provided the idea that the universe is a vast musical instrument, Human BioAcoustics provides the idea that the body is a mathematical universe that adheres to the principles that Pythagoras taught.

Studies conducted by my non-profit Institute of BioAcoustic Biology and Sound Health have consistently demonstrated that math can be much more than a measurement tool. The case studies my fellow researchers and I have amassed, using math as frequency-based biomarkers, indicate that the solution to therapeutic predictability and resolution has the potential to be a matter of frequency-based mathematical equations. This has been demonstrated in cases of severe allergic reactions, drug overdose, pain resolution, accelerated bone restructuring, heart arrhythmia, muscle and nerve atrophy, stroke recovery, sports trauma predictions, and more.

The body contains hundreds, if not thousands, of mathematical relationships. For example, the Human BioAcoustic frequency for the diabetes gene is the same frequency as a specific protein for the lens of the eye. This could potentially explain why diabetes and vision issues often appear together. Could both conditions be mathematically cured concurrently? Could reducing biology to a math-based framework give additional knowledge that simple symptom diagnostics cannot provide?

Although still in its early stages, this new science that is exploring this last lasting human conundrum appears to be on its way to being unveiled. My Institute's research has provided a foundation which demonstrates that just as there are chemical pathways of compounds, there are "Mathways" of subtractive frequencies that can be used to create numeric biomarker matrices capable, individually, and collectively, of being therapeutically predictive, diagnostic and prescriptive.

Mathematical relationships become apparent when a deeper dive into the math of medications is undertaken.

My aim and life purpose has always been to share this information with the public so that a nearly unlimited map of sound frequency formulations can be made available to the populace. To date, there is no universally accepted modality that has the potential to assist in our biological survival in the face of biological, radioactive, and pandemic threats, and the growing epidemic of chronic degenerative diseases. Using math in this way allows for an intrinsic evaluation of nutrients and biochemicals in a unique way, one that uses octaves of mathematical music scales to peer well below simple serum levels of conventional medicine blood, urine, and saliva tests. We actively take a sixteen-layer-deep view that helps discern the root cause of a person's health problems. Conventionally, in many instances, by the time the root cause of an issue has been identified, it is often too late to provide remediation.

Using the unique techniques of Vocal Profiling and evaluation, underlying, and often atypical emotional, as well as physiological, issues can be unraveled and resolved. The goal is to actively teach individuals and wellness providers to understand the freedoms created by the potential of Math as Medicine. Studies substantiate that the human voice can reveal data which indicates that people who share similar traumas, stress, diseases, and toxicities also share similar, if not identical, vocal anomalies. The data brings together ancient knowledge with modern ideas of harmonics and frequency relationships to show that math can be used as a form of predictive, diagnostic and curative therapy to support and enhance optimal wellness. Through entrainment of the frequency grid of the brain, the body can be programmed to support its own optimal form and function if the basic understanding of individual math-based homeostasis can be gleaned. The essential element is accurately identifying the appropriate, significant frequencies associated with each desired outcome. Human BioAcoustics makes all of this possible.

Conclusion

Just as a rainbow is incomplete without its full spectrum of colors, the human body needs full spectrum sounds that are created by the corresponding harmonic sets to establish and maintain a perfect state of health. The modern day principles of Human BioAcoustics and the ancient principles observed by Pythagoras have successfully been united to create a new science of Human BioAcoustic Biology. Emerging is a new science that recognizes the body's structure and function as a mathematical harmonic matrix. Repeatable studies have shown that human biology and interactions conform to a prescribed set of Body Harmonics. The new science will most certainly help to set the standards for the medicine of the future.

If we can influence our brains to heal us individually through the presentation of frequency-layered patterns of math – and we have proven that we can in many instances – why not explore that opportunity?

CHAPTER 4

THE SELF-HEALING BODY AND HUMAN BIOACOUSTIC BIOLOGY AS A VIABLE COMPONENT OF INTEGRATIVE MEDICAL DIAGNOSTICS AND TREATMENT

This chapter further explains the science that supports the use of Human BioAcoustics, as well as the underlying mechanisms of action that make its many benefits possible.

Over the decades that I've spent pioneering field of Human BioAcoustic Biology and using the voice as a mathematical matrix, I've been able to model the frequencies and architecture of human vocalizations to identify the innate numeric templates of the human body. Using the idea that the voice is a holographic representation of health and wellness, these non-invasive techniques are being advanced to the extent that a computerized Vocal Profile, using a system of Frequency Equivalents, can be used to accurately quantify, organize, interpret, define and extrapolate biometric information from the human voice.

This information, in turn, provides the opportunity to predict, direct, and maintain the intrinsic form and function of the body.

This novel approach has provided an accumulation of significant data that, until recently, has been without an efficient biological framework of reference. The lack of a scientifically-based foundational theory of Human BioAcoustics has prevented the field from moving forward as quickly as one might expect. Although the research results are impressive, historians will likely look at what has been accomplished to date as rudimentary.

The emerging model of "Math as Medicine," which I shared with you in Chapter 3, and which is being assembled from Human BioAcoustic research data, has the potential to allow voice spectral analysis to be used to predict health issues from the very first cries of a newborn through the frequency solutions of disease and aging.

Vocal Profiling can be used as a tool to identify and interpret the dynamic, complicated frequency interactions within the body. These techniques have provided insight into the possibility that the math-based biomarkers contained in the vocal patterns present a holographic representation of the human body.

Human BioAcoustics can most aptly be described as a cross between music therapy and biofeedback. It is related to music inasmuch as specific combinations of sounds are presented to elicit brain entrainment, but not necessarily sounds that would be considered musical.

To recap what you've read in previous chapters, some of the successful applications of Human BioAcoustics include:

1) monitoring of nutrients and food requirements from an internal perspective to support optimal cellular health
2) evaluation of weak and strong muscles to optimize physical strength and stamina
3) pre-screening for indications of disease, stress, and trauma
4) determination of bioterrorist substances and toxins in their genomic state before they become pathogenic, and
5) the solution to muscle atrophy and bone deterioration, including muscle atrophy and bone deterioration that is a serious threat to astronauts during space exploration.

Vocal Profiling has the potential to determine the biometric frequencies designed to diagnose and provide dominion over optimal form and function in the body. This is what explains how the health benefits achieved in the case histories that you read about in previous chapters, as well as the ones that follow in Chapter 5, came about.

When we consider the prospect of a medical paradigm shift that results in the ability to use the voice as a self-diagnostic tool to manage and restore health biologically through the entrainment of cells from the inside out, we quickly realize that the potential and implications are staggering. Our biggest issue, if this new paradigm shift occurs, is verified, and accepted, will be what to do with all the resources and time we now spend on our health. Imagine what could be accomplished if the $4+ trillion that the United States pays annually towards health care could be used instead for other equally important issues facing our nation.

The Emergence of Vocal Profiling As A Self-Diagnostic Tool

From thousands of case studies conducted by more than 200 trained Human BioAcoustic Research Associates, the concept of the human voice as a mathematical matrix of the body has been recognized and verified to be a useful, accurate, and elegant method for examining the architecture and frequency environments associated with the numerical pathways of human biology and physiology. These predictable cascades are now being used to identify the signature pathways of complex disease states.

Vocal Profiling originated from my understanding, based on my innate, God-given ability, that the brain generates and receives impulse patterns that can be measured through voice spectral analysis. These frequency impulses serve as directives to sustain the body's structural integrity, as well as maintaining emotional equilibrium. When these patterns are disrupted the brain seeks to alert the body by manifesting symptoms that are interpreted as disease and stress.

Vocal Profiling proves what I first began to realize as a child: the body requires the presence of a full range of harmonious frequencies working cooperatively in order to be healthy. Even in childhood, I could tell if a person was or was about to become sick if the frequencies their bodies emitted, and which I could perceive, were not in harmony and/or if one or more of the frequency notes of their Signature Sound (see Chapter 2) were missing. Since those around me during those years could not understand my abilities, it caused me a good degree of consternation, yet even then I knew what I was perceiving was true and correct. Invariably, those I encountered with inharmonious or missing frequencies were or became sick. But when I innocently stated such things as a child, I was often censured. Some people even thought I was possessed, so I soon learned to keep my mouth shut.

Fortunately, though, I never doubted or shut down my ability, and eventually, as an adult, once I gained a better understanding of it, I devoted myself to creating Human BioAcoustics and its Vocal Profiling system that it is my sincere wish will soon become more widely known and accepted because of the benefits it can provide to so many people around the world.

Consider the body as a musical instrument. When even one note is out of tune, the result is often discordant. Yet, when we tune the instrument, its sounds again become harmonious.

At present, only the number of practitioners and the acceptance, or lack of acceptance, by insurance underwriters, limits the scope and practice of Vocal Profiling. But now that computerization has allowed Human BioAcoustic assessment to become a complementary tool to conventional wellness practices, these improvements in assessment time and presentation delivery have the potential to allow Human BioAcoustic Profiling to become a standard diagnostic tool in doctors' offices, medical clinics, and hospitals around the world.

Just as importantly, because anyone who undergoes adequate training in Human BioAcoustics can become a Human BioAcoustic practitioner (you will learn how to do so in Chapter 9), the potential for this technology to be provided by people from all walks of life leads me to envision a day when it is available in every community, and even in every home. That is my most fervent hope and dream.

The benefits of this type of effective and accurate analytical tool could provide immediate, non-invasive medical modeling for predictive, diagnostic, and prescriptive consideration worldwide. Targeted techniques would include, but not be limited to:

Remote diagnoses and treatment
Assessment of nutritional requirements
Evaluation of environmental toxins
Screening for invading pathogen exposure
Appraisal of genetic syndromes
Diagnosis and evaluation of biochemical and metabolic conditions
Muscle strength and weakness status
Pre-vaccination risk factors analysis
Medication compatibility confirmation.

Now imagine being able to provide all of these services in your local community. The training curriculum I've developed, which I discuss in Chapter 9, make that possible today.

The Scientifically Proven Benefits of Vocal Profiling and Human BioAcoustics

Various studies using low-frequency analog sound presentation based on groups of people with similar traits and conditions have demonstrated the effectiveness of Human BioAcoustics for helping to resolve the following specific issues:
Bone and muscle concerns such as stress, strain, strength and trauma
Attention deficit disorder (ADD)
Macular degeneration
Infertility and pregnancy issues
Post traumatic stress disorder (PTSD)

Traumatic brain injury (TBI)

Parkinson's disease

Toxin exposure

Autism

Gout

Metabolic disorders

Arrhythmia and pre-vaccination risk factors

Epstein-Barr virus (EBV) and Chlamydia pneumonia exposure and identification.

In addition, double blind studies, laboratory tests, and studies based on comatose individuals, newborns, and mentally challenged persons have further established an evidence-based protocol for the study and use of biofrequencies.

Although the foundational principles of Human BioAcoustics continue to evolve, the results are undeniable. Based on existing research, it appears that sound presentation not only creates entrainment of brainwave frequencies, but that these frequencies also act as a support to the body until the body can maintain the required frequencies independently.

How Frequency, as Sound, Influence Bodily Form and Function

It is well known, historically, that sound and rhythms have the ability to influence mood and behavior. Literature published in the field of music therapy is replete with data which proves that frequency in the forms of music, rhythm, resonance, vibration, magnetics, etc., can influence the body in a myriad of different and dramatic ways.

This is obvious and can be witnessed through predictable adrenaline responses to potentially dangerous sounds, and to our hormonal responses to sexually explicit suggestions. We use sound to soothe our infants and then throughout life to stimulate and entertain. At the end of life, funeral services are accompanied by dirges that have been expressly written to help the survivors move through grief.

While a great deal of the response to sound is learned, it is commonly understood that human newborns will demonstrate a startle reflex to loud, unfamiliar sounds. Not only does the human infant unconsciously respond, but newborn animals also respond to unknown or startling sounds as part of their survival instincts. Animals, like humans, learn to ignore habituated sound. Research also demonstrates that animals and plants respond differently to different types of music.

Sound, music, rhythm and song are all used to create mood for entertainment purposes. There are books written with listings of which songs and note combinations elicit specific emotions. The late Candace Pert skillfully concluded in her revolutionary book, *Molecules of Emotion*, that a biological relationship exists between the body and mind. Her research clearly demonstrated that sensory influences shape the biochemical and structural characteristics of the human body. In particular, peptide-based proteins were identified by her as the "molecules of emotion".

Sounds have the ability to make your skin prickle, make your knees weak, make you perspire, cause the heart to beat in an irregular fashion, cause loss of control of the bladder, cause you to be sad, tense, excited, happy, or peaceful, to name just a few of the ways we respond to sound. The sensory input of sound via voice, music, noise, and rhythms has a demonstrated influence on the form and function of the body. Probably one of the most common examples of this phenomenon is the hormonal change that a teenage boy experiences as he moves through puberty. These changes certainly have an influence on his voice as it changes during his journey into adulthood.

The Universe as Frequency: Science has long held the model of the Universe as being frequency based. Our world is in a state of constant oscillation. Everything is vibrating. We interpret these vibrations through our senses, but each pulsation reaches the brain as a frequency representation. When the eye perceives the frequency vibrations of light, the eye changes those vibrations into electrical-chemical energy (another form of frequency) and sends those frequency impulses to the brain. The brain, receiving the information as frequency, routes that range of frequency to the appropriate area of the brain to interpret the input as visual data. The same sequence of events takes place when we are exposed to aromas, auditory input, tactile stimulation, emotional situations and so on.

Ancient, as well as modern, religious practices also incorporate sound (frequency), vibration, and rhythm into their rituals of worship. Science dictates that the lowest common denominator of all structure, the atom, is energy, which can be measured as frequency. Therefore, from our beliefs to our physical reality, frequency is the basis of our universe.

Essentially all forms of curative intervention influence the frequency systems of the body. There are many forms of medical acoustics: X-rays, sonograms, ultrasounds, MRIs, CAT scans, TENS units, etc. One of the most common medical devices based on frequency medicine is the heart pacemaker.

We are slowly learning to use frequency to help the body diagnose and heal itself. When we learn the governing patterns of each person's individual frequency signatures, we are able to interpret and have control over all aspects of our bodies' mechanical and biochemical conditions and often our emotional issues, as well.

As I've discussed earlier in this book, the techniques of Human BioAcoustics have the ability to record the frequencies of the body via the voice and to then return those frequencies using low-frequency ambient sound. Joseph Fourier demonstrated that the frequencies of the human voice could be expressed as mathematical algorithms. Vocal sounds are made possible by the oscillations of the vocal cords located in the voice box or larynx. The muscles of the larynx are innervated by branches of the laryngeal nerve, which is a branch of the vagus nerve. The vagus nerve is the 10th cranial nerve and is responsible for the sensations of the larynx which is the main nerve of the parasympathetic nervous system.

Through the entrainment of the vagus nerve with the vocal cords, a direct message pathway from the vocal cords and the brain seems apparent. The sounds of the voice, therefore, can be seen as representations of the parasympathetic nervous system. Together, the sympathetic and para-sympathetic nerve branches monitor and manage body functions.

Frequency As Language: Our brain communicates using the language of math expressed as frequency. The brain receives and assigns signals to specific areas for interpretation and possible reactions. Everything that happens to the body reaches the brain as a biofrequency that is then sorted, routed, and assigned an interpretation designation. Our brain uses a network of frequencies to internally communicate. We use a network of vocal sounds (and gestures) to communicate externally. Both are ranges of frequency, nerve impulses, and the voice respectively. When we speak, our vocal cavity vibrates, setting up a resonance that can be felt in many structures of the body. These resonant frequencies have a dramatic influence on the body as we speak and listen.

This dual incoming and outgoing frequency exchange of the voice and ears can be used to evaluate and interpret the frequency relationships within the body to represent who we are, our health and our well-being. This identifying frequency is called a Signature Sound (see Chapter 2) by many schools of ancient thought. It is actually a combination of frequencies and could be more accurately described as a Signature Octave or Chord.

There is also an identifying sound that can be measured through the ear canal. It is called the oto-acoustic emission. Much has been written about this phenomenon, particularly by Guy Berard, MD, the original inventor of Auditory Integration Training. (AIT). He found that the ear has a full range of frequencies which can be monitored, recorded, and retrained. The effect of this auditory retraining can bring about the reversal of diseases such as autism.

The idea of Human BioAcoustics and other types of sound therapy is simple and effective: Change the frequency and the body responds by eliminating dysfunction and disease.

James Cowan reported in the journal *Environmental Acoustics* that the ear canal is, on average, a tube about 1.2 inches in length, depending on a person's age and physiology. The size of the ear canal, which is open on one end and closed by the eardrum on the other, actually resembles a pipe organ and can resonate between 2700 and 3500 Hz (that equates to the notes of F through A in modern American music). Since the tubular structure of the ear is only capable of creating a small portion of the entire musical scale, it is obvious that oto-acoustic emissions are created somewhere other than the ear canal itself.

This individually identifying frequency emission is measurable and has been studied extensively by Dorinne Davis. Davis has cross-referenced Human BioAcoustic Vocal Profiling with oto-acoustic emissions in a study of a heterogeneous group of subjects (people with dissimilar characteristics). She found that 100 percent of the subjects had oto-acoustic emissions that specifically matched an identified point on the vocal print as being a stressed frequency.

This is statistically relevant when you consider that 100,000 frequencies are considered but a Human BioAcoustic vocal scan only chooses up to 24 possible points as significant. When the results of Human BioAcoustic research were combined with the ongoing studies carried out by Davis with oto-acoustic emissions, it was obvious that both the ears and the voice have the ability to identify frequencies of stress.

Although Human BioAcoustic research has yet to substantiate this, consideration should be given to the possibility that we learn to derive meaning from ambient sound by interruptions in the oto-acoustic emissions. Much like a pebble dropped into still water, sound wave interruptions send a binary signal that is assigned meaning through past experience.

How Frequency Expressed As Vibration Influences the Body According To Scientists

It's now widely accepted that frequency vibrations influence the body, with the effects varying depending on the frequency. How does this happen?

To answer that question, James L. Oschman, PhD, a leading investigator of biophysics and energy medicine offers this explanation:

"At an atomic scale, physical contact between two molecules has less meaning than the ways they interact energetically. As a hormone approaches a receptor, the electronic structures of both molecules begin to change. Bonds bend, twist and stretch; parts rotate and wiggle. The orientation and shape of the molecules change so that the active site of the hormone can approach the active site of the receptor. The recognition of a specific hormone by a receptor depends on resonant vibratory interactions, comparable to the interactions of tuning forks."

Oschman further states that "the rotation of a charged amino acid sets up an electromagnetic field that entrains rotations of the corresponding amino acid on a second protein. The second protein also emits an electromagnetic field that affects other proteins."

Oschman specifically cited the Diapulse device as an example of this. The Diapulse emits 27 MHz and has been extensively researched. Clinical trials show that the Diapulse can reduce swelling, accelerate wound healing, stimulate nerve regeneration, and reduce pain due to the frequency vibrations it emits. This demonstrates that biochemicals communicate, and that external frequencies have a healing influence. The quandary then becomes the identification of the avenue by which the body prompts these internal healing frequencies.

Oschman referenced the work of K.J. Pienta and D. D. Coffery from their 1991 paper entitled "Cellular Harmonic Information Transfer through a Tissue Tensigrity-Matrix System" to prove the point that the body dynamically communicates via a frequency based matrix. He stated, "Cells and intracellular elements are capable of vibrating in a dynamic manner with complex harmonics, the frequency of which can now be measured and analyzed in a quantitative manner by Fourier analysis... These vibrations can be altered by growth factors and the process of carcinogenesis. It is important to understand the mechanism by which this vibrational information is transferred directly throughout the cell...The vibrational interactions occur through a tissue matrix system consisting of the nuclear matrix, the cytoskeleton, and the extracellular matrix that is poised to couple the biological oscillations of the cell from the peripheral membrane to the DNA through a tensegrity-matrix system."

The late Valerie Hunt, Ed.D., Professor Emeritus at UCLA, and a respected neurophysiologist and author of several books on the subject of bioenergy, was a pioneer in the field of human energy fields. She believed that all living systems are composed of vibrations, which organize themselves into fields as we interact with our environment, our emotions and other people. Her research revealed a direct correlation between healing and the vibrational rates of human energy fields. For those of you who find the idea of an energy field a bit esoteric, please note that without energy your body would be inert. The body's energy field animates your every move.

The late scientist William Tiller, PhD, Chairman of Stanford's Materials Science Department, carried out extensive research based upon the vibrational signals of the body. He wrote, "Each atom and molecule, cell and gland in our body has a characteristic frequency at which it will both absorb and emit radiation." Each cell generates its own minute vibrational signals from within that must stay in resonance with every other cell for the body to remain healthy.

Two Cornell University physics graduate students, Barry Stripe and Mohammad Rezaei, reported in the June 1998 issue of *Science* that each atom has an identifying "energy level" that can be used to identify individual molecules and unknown chemicals by measuring their vibrational signatures.

These are but a few examples of how distinguished scientists and researchers have discovered and explained the effects of frequencies and vibrations on the body right down to the cellular and atomic level. From many fields of study, both conceptual and established, the premise that the body is based on, responds to, and is influenced by frequency is increasingly becoming an accepted reality.

Entrainment Through Cellular Oscillation

The concept of entrainment in music is common. If one string of an instrument vibrates, the remaining strings will set up a resonant harmony with the original vibrating string. Metronomes set in motion manually will fall into temporal alignment. That is, they tend to perform their motions in sync with one another. When we take pleasure in music, our body begins to move in time with the rhythm. Hormonal entrainment has been observed among women who work together. One result of this is that their menstrual cycles will often synchronize.

Entrainment of the vocal cords by the vagus nerve is also an accepted physiological fact. The vagus nerve is the tenth of twelve cranial nerves that provide communication pathways from the lower organs to the brain. The vagus nerve is also responsible for sensory innervations from the larynx to the vocal cords and the motor signals that vibrate the vocal cords.

Vagus nerve therapy through implanted vagal nerve stimulators shows that stimulation of the vagus nerve changes the voice. Studies conducted at the University of Chicago Medical Center have shown that direct stimulation to the vagus nerve can prevent seizures known to be caused by chaotic neuron firings in the brain.

The importance of speech signals to evaluate mental and physical status has long been used as a scientifically reliable method of objective assessment of psychophysiological stress, cardiovascular health, and aging.

The vagus nerve connection also lies within the province of philosophy and has been espoused by noted theosophist Alice Bailey. The ancient practices of yoga and Qigong teach that stimulation and relaxation of the vagus nerve is healthful, as well.

From esoteric philosophy to modern science, the connection between the vagus nerve and health has long been recognized as a reality. Yet, for much of that time no one knew how to quantify this information to allow for the development of an interactive, precise protocol for interpretation and use. Using voice spectral analysis to evaluate the physical and biochemical status of the body is a logical combination of using the vagus nerve via the vocal cords to convey internal information through an external source (the voice) for measurement.

Human BioAcoustics stands between these two realms of thought and is often accused of being too esoteric by the scientific field and too scientific by the philosophical genre. The domain of Human BioAcoustics exists as a combination of the inspired creativity of musical formats and the integrated scientific evaluation for health, wellness, and self-healing outcomes.

Sound, Music, and Mathematics As a Healing Modality: Using frequency in such forms as sound, color, music, and rhythm has long been an esoteric avenue to support physical and spiritual health. Paleoanthropologist Noel T. Boaz in his book *Eco Homo*, an investigation of human evolution and the natural history of our human origins, reported that the archeological evidence left by the Upper Paleolithic culture, which is estimated to have existed around 30,000 BC, indicates that these ancient musicians used flutes to match resonant frequencies found in caves.

As humans evolved, music developed into levels of intricate harmony nestled within structures of great elegance. Professor Susumu Ohno, of the Beckman Research Institute, proposed that musical composition and human DNA are both governed by the same patterns of repetition. He stated in science journal *Immunogenetics* that "the all pervasive principle of repetitious recurrence governs not only coding sequence construction but also human endeavor in musical composition." This is obvious to anyone listening to human DNA when it is converted mathematically to frequency sequences. The result sounds musical.

Dr. David Schwartz of Duke University in North Carolina has provided many clues as to how music and speech have evolved. His team of researchers found that the mathematical speech patterns of all languages cluster at the designated points assigned as the musical notes and scales of that particular culture.

Vocal Profiling has always emphasized the significance of the harmonic balance of notes of a scale relative to the study of Human BioAcoustics. To learn that independent researchers have found supporting evidence which further confirms the postulates of BioAcoustics is, indeed, refreshing.

Such convincing evidence shows that using sound to facilitate change within the body is an ancient perspective. Using sound to seek dominion over the body has been a cherished part of almost every human culture, but these efforts were often surrounded with superstition and mysticism. It wasn't until computer technology and instrumentation was developed to manage the massive amount of data required that the vibrational mathematics of the body could be used to individually diagnose and prescribe. Using the body's own sound system as a foundation, the ears and skin perceive sound, and the voice reproduces it.

Vibration Is To Brain Frequencies As Heart Is To Rhythm: Entrainment is also a concept used in Human BioAcoustics when ambient sound formulations are presented to a client.

The following is a graph that depicts three sets of synchronized oscillations. The heartbeat of the person being "toned to" is represented by the top line. The middle graph is the beat frequency of the tone being presented. The bottom line is the heartbeat of the person doing the toning. It is obvious that the hearts of both the toner and the person being toned to, have entrained to the tone represented by the middle line. The synchronization seems to be instantaneous when a competent toner begins to vocalize a sound.

Actual EKG Data - heart rhythms synchronized of a Toner, a tone and a person receiving tones

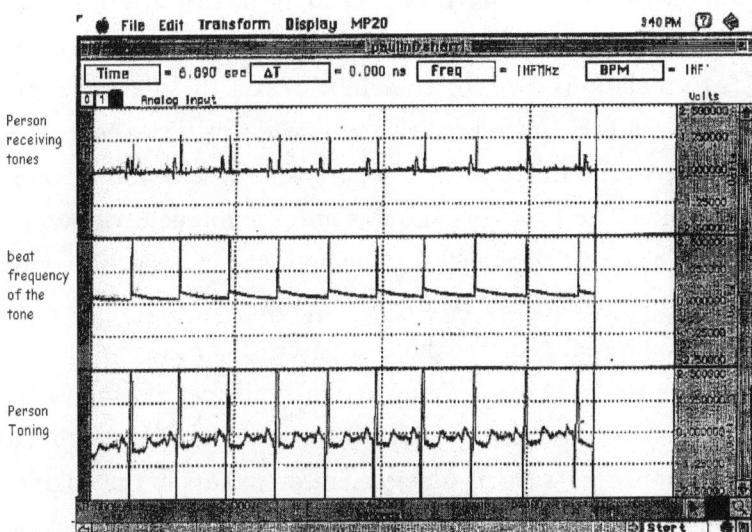

The next graph is of brain waves that were taken at the same time as the heartbeat entrainment data was gathered. The brain waves of both the toner and the person being toned to have synchronized, showing entrainment through the vocal presentation of ambient sound.

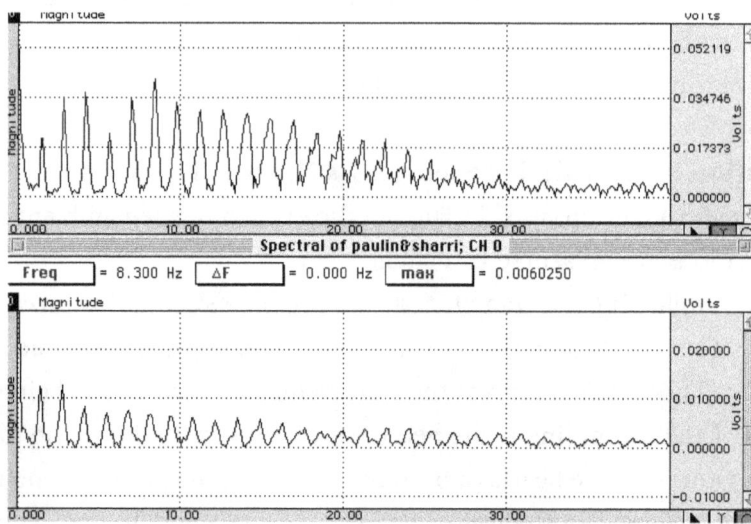

Human BioAcoustics uses this same principle. Specific frequency combinations entrain the brain waves, and the rhythm entrains the heart. When the heart and brain are functioning as one unit, healing is often the result. This has been extensively researched by the Institute of Heart Math located in Boulder Creek, California.

The formulations used for Human BioAcoustic sound presentation are triadic in nature. (In music, a triad is a set of three notes that can be stacked vertically in thirds. Triads are the most common chords in Western music.) The Frequency Equivalent is combined with an Energy Equivalent. These two frequencies are then united in a specific configuration that is presented for evaluation during tone trials.

This triadic sequence can be compared to preparing your car to drive. You are required to turn on the ignition (identify the Frequency Equivalent), engage the gear (the sequenced formulation combination), and, finally, apply pressure to the accelerator to supply the engine with fuel, which will ignite, to provide the power (the Energy Equivalent).

Intention as a Requirement for Entrainment: During experiments (including those mentioned above) that produced entrain ment, the concept of intention was considered. Below are voice wave forms of the same toner compared to normal vocal prints:

A wave form taken when the toner was asked to think about church bells.

A wave form when the toner was asked to think about and discuss a religious building.

A wave form taken as the toner was thinking about clasped fingers.

And finally a comparison of magnetic strip patterns and the toner's voice.

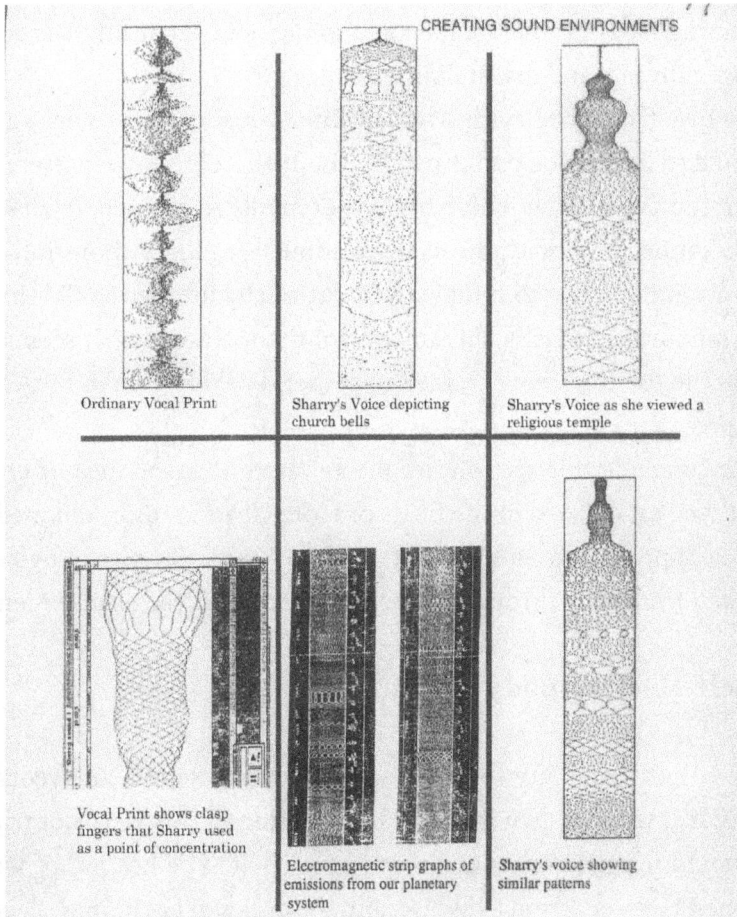

CREATING SOUND ENVIRONMENTS

Ordinary Vocal Print

Sharry's Voice depicting church bells

Sharry's Voice as she viewed a religious temple

Vocal Print shows clasp fingers that Sharry used as a point of concentration

Electromagnetic strip graphs of emissions from our planetary system

Sharry's voice showing similar patterns

Some of the above vocal prints are complex sine waves, something supposedly impossible for a human voice to produce. The mathematical configurations of these prints are the matrix principles upon which Human BioAcoustic formulations are based. These wave forms indicate that a toner can intentionally create a "sound image" using sine waves produced by the voice. This translates to the idea of intention as a component of healing and certainly needs further exploration.

An example of this was a young man who had been in a motorcycle accident which severely damaged his lower legs. One issue was his inability to lift the big toe of his right foot. Human BioAcoustic evaluation identified the Frequency Equivalent as being that assigned to the soleus muscle. (The soleus muscle is located in the back part of the lower leg, running from just below the knee to the heel. Its health is crucial for walking, running, and maintaining balance.)

Before treatment with Human BioAcoustics, the man valiantly attempted to lift the toe on his own without success. As we presented the ambient sounds without telling him, he excitedly responded, "I got it. I got it." The sound presentation was discontinued (again without informing him), causing him not to be able to intentionally lift the toe. With sound support, he was gradually able to control the toe muscles. It seems obvious that the toe was being trained to respond to the Human BioAcoustic sound presentation.

To conclude this section, let me reiterate that the idea of entrainment is well established in the fields of biofeedback, music, and medicine. Research supports the notion that the body responds physiologically to sound and frequency through the achievement of cyclic entrainment.

The Self-Healing Body

The body has the ability to self-diagnose, self-prescribe, and reorganize itself according to its own intrinsic information. If this were not true, the body would neither repair nor regenerate itself. The healing of wounds and bones, recovery from a disease, and the cycles of hormones, sleep, and hunger would be totally implausible. Certainly the idea of generating an entirely new human life during gestation would not be possible without a self-instructed, reproductive directive functioning independently within the biological terrain of the body.

Continuous networks of biological signals (biofrequencies) provide information and direction to produce and reproduce inherent form and function. Tapping into these self-healing biological pathways from brain to neuron to cell has long been a goal of scientific medical investigations as a way to provide and promote optimal health.

These observations are obvious, but who, or what, has dominion over these processes? Why has medical science not been able to completely access and explain this internal alchemy? In our limited wisdom, should we have access to knowledge of such potent significance? The answer may not be obvious, but it is inevitable. If such a unifying premise were to exist it would contain not only a diagnostic component but also a method of management and resolution.

If such an operative prescription for maintenance and renewal could be accessed, it would permit dominion over the innate processes of the body that are mandatory for rejuvenation, nutritional and structural requirements, appropriate detoxification systems, and potentially perpetual regeneration.

If, in addition, that system could predict how the body would react based on genomic, environmental, and internal stimuli, it would be an incredible advancement in the world of medicine. It is my contention that Human BioAcoustics, based on the accuracy of its diagnostic methods and its ability to significantly improve a wide range of health conditions via its delivery of appropriate frequencies, has the potential to be such a system.

The mathematical concepts used to construct Human BioAcoustic formulations (see Chapter 3) are associated with the Pythagorean theory of string harmonics. Today, modern string theorists postulate that the universe is made of uncountable, infinitesimal strings that group together to create matter. But those same scientists readily admit that they have inadequate information pertaining to how the strings actually create the DNA of life.

Science has proven that electrical nerve impulses are managed by magnetic potential. When examining the mathematical relationships of Human BioAcoustic Biology, it seems obvious that the interactions are being measured and managed by the magnetic resonance of sound harmonics. This could be seen as being akin to the management of the "Field" surrounding each cell and, in turn, each individual, as described by Bruce Lipton and Lynn McTaggart in their respective works, *Biology of Belief* and *The Field*.

Human BioAcoustic evaluation can predict the outcome of a frequency presentation which is turn indicates that Human BioAcoustic formulations may be the answer to the regulation of what is created by DNA strings. History may view Human BioAcoustic Biology as the move from a fractional to a quantum concept of health.

The Mechanics of Human BioAcoustics: Recapping what you learned in Chapter 1, the protocol for Human BioAcoustics is a two part process: Vocal Profiling and Sound Presentation. Vocal Profiling offers interpretative information and can stand independently as a valuable assessment tool. Sound presentation provides the management phase through brain wave entrainment using low-frequency, ambient sound.

A. Vocal Profiling

Using a computerized vocal sample, the frequencies and architecture of the voice are individually analyzed and used to create a multiple page report that can be used to examine the Frequency Equivalents (FE) of the biochemical pathways and physical structures of individual human biology. Report options include, but are not limited to: muscles, toxins, genes, proteins, pathogen exposure, biochemicals, nutrients, immune and metabolic issues, vaccination safety, and other risk factors, all of which are evaluated in terms of Frequency Equivalents.

Each report can be used by trained personnel to provide predictive and immediate, non–invasive information for individual health and medical management in term of FEs and brain wave entrainment. The vision for the future is to continue to create frequency templates using computers to automate the assessment. At present there are 1000's of biofrequency templates that have been organized into over 200 software template programs.

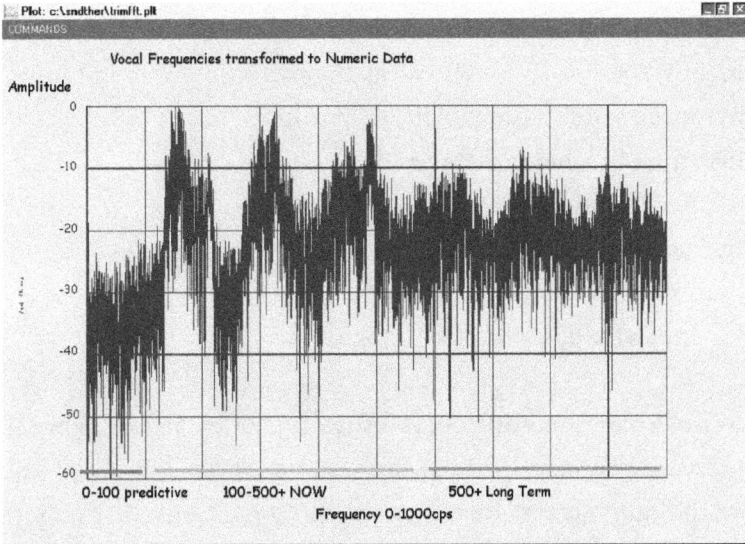

Vocal Fast Fourier Transform (FFT) showing Predictive, NOW and Long Term frequency ranges.

At present there are a range of options for predictive measurements which have been verified in an impressive number of case studies, and medical lab tests have verified the efficacy of Human BioAcoustic Frequency Equivalents.

Below is a Human BioAcoustic Frequency Equivalent Report of a volunteer. The computerized report indicated that a thyroid issue might be indicated. Medical lab reports ordered by the client's physician confirmed the Human BioAcoustic observations. After being prescribed the appropriate medications by his physician, the client reported increased energy, an improved sleeping routine, and memory improvement.

Thyroid Client #7-12
PROVIDER LISTING
The following Frequency Equivalents™ *have been identified*
DIR STATUS NAME CATEGORY
L Liothyronine Sodium Biochemical/thyroid
L Tri-Iodothyronine/T3 Biochemical/thyroid
L Liothyronine Biochemical/thyroid
S Tri-Iodothyronine/T3 Biochemical/thyroid
S Liothyronine sodium Biochemical/thyroid
S Liothyronine Biochemical/thyroid
S Thyroxine/T4 Hormone
L Liothyronine-T3 Hormone/thyroid
S Liothyronine-T3 Hormone/thyroid
[key; S = unbalanced; L = low; H = high]

Human BioAcoustics and Social Issues: Not only can biochemical issues be displayed by Human BioAcoustic vocal patterns, but social issues, or what we thought were social issues, are observable as well. For example:

Teenagers often build up an overabundant, intolerable level of the most common frequencies belonging to their parents. This would indicate that the recalcitrant behavior, about which nearly all parents complain, is actually a design of nature to separate parents and their children. The exception is the child who is of opposite brain dominance than the parents. This child will remain at home forever, if allowed.

A woman who has just been beaten by her mate will often go back to that companion if he has the frequencies that she needs to feel complete. Each person has a set of frequencies that are more and less abundant in their vocal print. When we meet someone with the same dominant notes, we may tend to clash with that person. When the new acquaintance has the frequencies we need, there may be an immediate attraction. It is mathematical as well as hormonal.

A frequency can represent a muscle as well as a compound. Women tend to admire broad shoulders, a strong chin, and a flat stomach. The Frequency

Equivalents responsible for the traits above are also the Frequency Equivalents of several male sex hormones. Are we attracted to the biological structure, or does the attraction come from the Frequency Equivalents of the male hormones which would indicate strong masculine genetic traits?

Human BioAcoustics and Biochemical Issues: Other biological issues often have mathematical implications that can be determined by Human BioAcoustic Vocal Profiling. For example:

Human BioAcoustics has shown a strong relationship between the measles vaccine and peripheral neuropathy (numbness in the hand and feet), autism and hepatitis, autism and zonulin, pertussis and bioflavonoids, vitamin A and autism, and polio with the SV40 vaccine and immune disorders.

The frequencies representing calcium and magnesium, when combined, produce the bone matrix protein. Calcium and magnesium are required for healthy bones.

Uric acid, which is associated with gout, and glucose are common factors for diabetics. Uric acid and glucose have a common mathematical matrix: A xanthine oxidase inhibitor is often prescribed for gout. Xanthine is involved in free radical production associated with diabetes.

Snoring is associated with diabetes and heart disease. The muscles that are involved in snoring have direct Frequency Equivalent associations with insulin and the biochemistry of the heart.

Anthrax pathogenic infiltration and the common cold have very similar Frequency Equivalents. They also have very similar initiating symptoms.

Etiocobalamin (a form of vitamin B12) and the vertical muscle of the tongue are not the same Frequency Equivalent, but they are nearly always found together within the charts of persons who have been diagnosed with Lou Gerhig's disease, both singly and in combination with Lyme Disease. In both cases the control of the tongue muscles are usually involved, and etiocobalamin seems to provide significant support for muscle strength and integrity.

The body produces hyaluronic acid using the amino acid proline and vitamin A. When one combines these two Frequency Equivalents the result is the Frequency Equivalent of hyaluronic acid.

Sexual response, or the lack thereof, can be traced mathematically to the pathway that is causing the reaction. Human BioAcoustic pilot studies have shown that libido can be increased by identifying and controlling sexual hormone response by the use of frequency presentations.

The Fireman's cough, which was common in many New York City 9/11 emergency workers, can be traced to a fire retardant that has the same Frequency Equivalent as the throat muscles. In addition the same Frequency Equivalent identifying the fire retardant relates to early onset breast cancer frequencies. Given more data, we might be able to predict that a higher incidence of early onset breast cancer will occur in the population surrounding New York City's Ground Zero.

There are 100,000 possible frequencies that can be chosen from a vocal print. Several times a gene that was decoded for a particular case study appeared among the 24 points pulled from a vocal print of a person who had been diagnosed with that particular gene stress.

Anecdotal though it may be, at least three people (including an RN and a MD) credit Human BioAcoustic sound presentations with stopping their episodes of anaphylactic shock from bee stings and allergic reactions.

In short, Human BioAcoustics has provided a foundation to substantiate that the mathematical matrix of FEs emulate the structure, genetic make-up, and biochemistry of the body.

B. BioAcoustic Sound Presentation

The autonomic nervous system, through its billions of neural interactions, is responsible for the monitoring, maintenance and stasis of every minute detail of our individual existence.

This regenerative process is not limited to sentient beings. Therefore, this course of development is not necessarily a feature of intention, advanced cognitive planning, or something that is under conscious control. If sexual intercourse occurs within the appropriate time frame, without preventative intervention, pregnancy will likely result. The body, independently, knows how to handle this biological feature. All creatures large and small, brained and brainless, reproduce in some way. If reproduction did not happen, that organism would cease to exist after one generation.

The actions and reactions of the autonomic nervous system are largely involuntary. So how does the body "know" how to act, how to regenerate, how to repair? What system is involved? Is it pure mechanics? Are we simply organic robots?

We humans, in our quest for qualitative and quantitative enlightenment, have divided the nervous system of the body into several layered branches, beginning with the peripheral nervous system and the central nervous system. The peripheral nervous system is further divided into the sensory-somatic nervous system and the autonomic nervous system. The autonomic nervous system consists of sensory neurons and motor neurons that run between the central nervous system and various organs.

The autonomic nervous system is divided into the parasympathetic and sympathetic nervous systems. These two regulatory agents monitor and regulate the actions and reactions of the body.

Sympathetic Versus Parasympathetic
(Spinal pathways) (Vagus nerve)
Stimulates heartbeat/Slows down heartbeat
Raises blood pressure/Lowers blood pressure
Dilates the pupils/Constriction of the pupils
Shunts blood away from skin/Increases blood flow to skin
Inhibits peristalsis in GI tract/Causes peristalsis of the GI tract.

When we anticipate eating a favorite dessert, the sympathetic system stimulates saliva in anticipation of receiving the dessert. The body is so adaptive that it will recognize which variety of enzyme is required by the expected sweet even before we experience the first morsel.

The body responds to unusual stimuli through the sympathetic nervous system. Responses to loud, non-habituated sounds normally produce an excretion of adrenaline to prepare the body for an unfamiliar event. A person can learn to sleep near a loud train railway and not be awakened by the noise, but not all responses to sound are learned. A baby, even a baby animal, has an instinctual reflex to loud noises. Even if the noise is familiar, hearing it at an unexpected interval can cause a startle response.

The parasympathetic nervous system is regulated through the vagus nerve which also regulates the motor impulses of the vocal cords. The vagus nerve through the spinal cord has a direct pathway to the brain. Through entrainment of the vocal cords and the vagus nerve, the sounds produced by the vocal cords can be perceived as a holographic representation of the regulating parasympathetic nervous system.

Biological Entrainment: The central nervous system (CNS) is an interactive "intranet" that allows constant information from millions of body processes to collaborate. This is what keeps our bodies functioning as an inclusive unity of atoms, cells, tissues, organs, and systems. The majority of these activities unite with the brain through the twelve cranial nerves. The vagus nerve, in particular, plays a significant role in these processes.

Human BioAcoustics offers a glimpse into the mathematical modeling and understanding of that CNS process through entrainment of the vagus nerve to the vocal cords. Since the vagus nerve is a direct pathway to the brain, and the vocal cords lie within the structures of the vagus nerve bundle, the voice can be perceived as a direct frequency representation of the sympathetic and parasympathetic expressions of the body.

Ongoing studies have shown that changing the timing of the frequency formulation protocols used in Human BioAcoustics allows organs to be directly targeted for intervention. Using a vocal sample in comparison to the known principles of the body's mathematical matrix allows frequency intervention to support the intrinsic conduct of self-healing.

Through Human BioAcoustics, the self-healing is often perceived as being so natural that people sometimes insist that it was just time for the body to get well on its own. A video demonstration of the management of gout pain by manipulating the body's frequency antidote for gout shows the absolute dominion over gout pain using Human BioAcoustic sound presentation. The video shows an MD who was experiencing the pain, redness, and swelling of gout, as the symptoms were provoked and then eliminated. This was repeated several times in the same session by the presentation and withdrawal of frequencies known to support the body in dealing with the symptoms of this very painful type of arthritis.

This influence of the body's ability to respond to low frequency sound has repeatedly been demonstrated. Case study videos showing the testing of muscle strength and weakness; the stimulation of B12 to increase strength and stamina; the control of adrenaline related behaviors in children; and the dominion over muscle related trauma and stress (multiple sclerosis for instance), all provide ample proof that Human BioAcoustic brain wave entrainment can positively influence the structure and function of the body.

Biofeedback is used to identify appropriate frequency combinations for the body. Using low frequency ambient sound, the client is asked to experience the sounds for specific amounts of time and to report their responses. Reassessment is essential to ensure that the sounds are being used for the appropriate amount of time.

The presentation of Frequency Equivalents seems to be akin to ingesting a vitamin. It is not the vitamin that achieves the healing; it is what the body does with the vitamin that makes the difference. The same is true of what the body does with the Frequency Equivalents.

The Voice As A Holographic Representation of the Body: The voice, as sung as music, is a calculated mathematical arrangement of sounds. The voice as spoken language is a complex, yet often mathematically chaotic, conglomeration of sounds. Each word is made up of individual sound units called phonemes. Human BioAcoustics examines the chaos and the disharmony of these phonemes. The foundational principle on which Human BioAcoustics has been established is the concept that the voice is a holographic representation of the body. The frequencies, the coherence patterns, and the architecture of the voice have been used to develop a computerized technology that can provide a glimpse into the individual, mathematical patterns that make up the body.

Steven Xue, Ph.D., a noted researcher in the arena of the voice and health, has shown a definitive relationship between the voice, health, and aging. Xue studied the role of 21 vocal changes in relationship to health, such as the role of sleep apnea and snoring as it relates to vocal sound waves. In an interview, Xue reiterated the importance of understanding which vocal changes are normal and which may signal health problems.

Danielle Campbell-Angah, editor of *ADVANCE for Audiologists and Speech Pathologists*, states that the quality of nutrients ingested has a significant impact on vocal health. Campbell explains, "On a cellular level the body depends on specific nutrients for the best performance of each individual cell. In this same way certain enzymes, co-enzymes, vitamins and minerals have an effect on the functioning of the vocal mechanism."

Rita Holl, in a 1996 article in *Alternative Health Practitioner*, hypothesized that the vocal prints of clients who had been diagnosed as having osteoarthritis and/or osteoporosis would demonstrate stress in the frequency equivalents assigned to calcium and magnesium (N=26).

Voice Analysis (Vocal Profiling) is much more than listening for allophones – a phonetic variation of a word that would differentiate the speech patterns of persons who might have a Texan or French accent. Human BioAcoustic computerization examines the biometric principles of the frequencies contained in the voice and then relates those patterns to an emerging mathematical matrix that is being assembled using several thousand case studies as a base.

Lab tests, and double blind, long term, and homogeneous case studies have all provided useful information that has worked to substantiate the voice as a multidimensional representation of the body.

Conclusion

My intention for this chapter is to present information that solidifies a foundational theory which will explain the obvious influences of sound, voice, rhythm, and song as a format to manage and support optimal human form and function through Human BioAcoustic evaluation and entrainment using low frequency sound presentation.

Ongoing research concerning voice spectral analysis and the presentation of individualized sound frequency formulations continues to demonstrate that Human BioAcoustics supports inherent health and wellness, often when other health interventions have failed. This innovative, ground-breaking field of study has utilized Vocal Profiling and low frequency analog sound presentation to reveal an inherent mathematical matrix in support of the self-healing body. This novel approach has provided an accumulation of impressive evidence that is staggering in its implications for Self-Health Care.

CHAPTER 5

NEW HOPE FOR THE HOPELESS— CASE HISTORIES THE DEMONSTRATE THE FULL SCOPE AND POWER OF HUMAN BIOACOUSTICS THERAPY TO HEAL

"Some day in the future, people will be cured
by sounds. It will be very practical."

~ Master healer Anthelme Nizier Phillipe de Lyon, 1898

I n this chapter I am going to share with you actual cases histories of some of my clients who recovered from a variety of health issues after receiving Human BioAcoustic Therapy. My purpose in sharing their stories is to further illustrate the breadth of benefits that Human BioAcoustics can provide.

In order to understand how these benefits are possible, please review Chapters 3 and 4.

Adrienne's Story

This first case history is about a young woman named Adrienne, and is recounted in his own words by her father, Robert Rodgers, PhD, founder of Parkinson's Recovery, an organization that provides information, support, and resources to people experiencing Parkinson's disease.

"I've had the pleasure of being a colleague of Sharry Edwards for many years. She's really a revolutionary in every respect. And when you really look at sound therapy, that is not therapies through medicines and surgeries, but rather therapies through sound, I really think that Sharry is the true pioneer in this entire field of technology.

"The best report that I can make about Sharry's work is the one that I'm most familiar with: What Sharry was able to do for my daughter Adrienne.

"For 20 years, Adrienne experienced periodic pain episodes that were so intense they caused a debilitating state of vomiting. Her pain was just off the charts and nothing really helped. During those years, she went to the ER approximately 70 times, where the medical staff would prescribe one opiate or anti-vomiting medication after another. Sometimes the drugs might provide a little bit of relief, but overall none of them were really useful. Adrienne tried everything, and nothing really cut the pain. She would be in the ER and be administered some IV hydration for about eight hours or more, sometimes a whole day, and then she'd be better. She could walk, she could function. But when she was discharged and her pain episodes returned, she could not walk. She couldn't function. She couldn't talk. At times, she couldn't even reason.

"It was just the most bizarre situation imaginable. Over time, her episodes of pain became very frequent and would last as long as three full days. I had been with her during several of those episodes where she just could not experience even the slightest degree of relief. The episodes became so frequent that she started calling me every other night saying, 'I can't do this. I don't want to be alive. There's no answer out there. Nobody has any solutions.' She eventually wound up being hospitalized for four months, seeing one set of doctors and specialists after another. They all did the best they could to try to figure out what was going on with Adrienne, and what kind of therapies might help provide her with some relief. She went through a lot of different specialists and a lot of different therapies and different drugs, yet she was not getting better. She was getting worse and worse.

"Thing reached the point to where I received a call from the medical team at the hospital. They reported to me that they tried everything to no avail, and recommended that it would probably be best for Adrienne to go into a hospice and nursing kind of a situation because they didn't think it would be beneficial for her to continue being treated at the hospital, since nothing they were doing for her was really helping. They didn't know what was wrong, but they were not optimistic about any kind of a positive outcome. So they asked for my permission to send her to a nursing home.

"I said, 'No, I'm sorry, but that doesn't work for me. She's young. We'll be able to figure out a solution.' So I took her out of the hospital and brought her home.

"I finally realized that I needed to look at this situation from a different perspective, since the medical professionals had done the best they could to figure out what they could do to help and support Adrienne, yet none of what they had to offer was helping.

"It was at that point that I considered the possibility that, if I sent Sharry some voice prints of Adrienne, she might be able to help. So Sharry began to work on Adrienne's voice prints and analyzed what it was that she saw. Interestingly, although Sharry told me that usually it doesn't take long to analyze a voice print to determine what's going on with them, with Adrienne she said she really had to dig very deeply and look at a lot different corners of her research world to figure out what was causing Adrienne's problems. Sharry worked intensively for a full week or more trying to find the answer.

"Another aspect of Adrienne's symptoms was that when she would experience the pain episodes, she would shake and exhibit tremors, just like people with Parkinson's disease, but it never occurred to me that there was any link between her condition and PD, despite all of the research I'd done on Parkinson's. Nor had I ever mentioned Adrienne's tremors to Sharry.

"Yet Sharry, on her own, began to explore this possibility, and was able to identify that Adrienne suffered from a very rare condition called dopamine-beta hydroxylase deficiency. Now, that's a mouthful, but its symptoms were exactly what Adrienne had been experiencing for many years: vomiting, dehydration, hypotension. hypothermia (she was always cold), and hypoglycemia. It is the first time we'd had any understanding of what was causing Adrienne's debilitating episodes.

"Sharry suggested that I tell Adrienne's medical doctor what she suspected might be at play with Adrienne to see if the hospital could confirm it with medical tests. So I shared Sharry's report with Adrienne's doctor, who agreed to look into it. She made quite a bit of effort looking to see what kind of test could they run for Adrienne to be able to determine whether or not Sharry's suspicion was valid, including conferring with a neurologist on her team. But she then called me to say they had not been able to identify any tests to be able to confirm Sharry's finding, and that she and the other doctors she'd consulted 'really don't know anything about this.'

"At that point, Sharry, again, very generously, crafted a set of 21 different sounds and placed them on a tone box for Adrienne. I also purchased a special speaker to connect the tone box to because that gives the sounds to the full body. This type of speaker is able to transmit very low frequency sounds. Sounds that we oftentimes, in an auditory sense, cannot even hear.

"The first process in terms of what needed to happen was that Adrienne listened to each of the tones separately. Sharry gave us very specific instructions to simply have Adrienne begin to listen to each tone, and to look for signs that it was either comforting to her or if it was causing some distress. I sat with Adrienne and watched her expressions and her breathing as she listened to each sound frequency. There was only one sound she had a little issue with, which we identified for Sharry. Sharry then programmed all of these tones together in one set of combined sounds and instructed Adrienne to listen to them each night when she was sleeping.

"Sharry also created a second set of sounds that were designed to be played whenever Adrienne realized that one of her pain episodes was coming on. And so we did all that, and Adrienne began getting a little better every day. Not huge or remarkable improvements, but we could see that things were shifting in the right direction.

"After several weeks, I recorded an updated voice print, but this time from when Adrienne had another one of her episodes. She could barely talk, but we went ahead and recorded the voice print and sent it to Sharry. Sharry did some updated analyses and found some additional issues. One of them turned out to be a Lyme disease infection, which Adrienne thought that she'd had for a number of years, but nobody had ever been able to help address that problem.

"Sharry reprogrammed the tone box and sent it back to Adrienne, who began to listen to the new tones. The result is that Sharry's Human BioAcoustic sound therapy proved to be a godsend for my daughter Adrienne. For the first time, we have an approach that is helping Adrienne heal. As she continued listening to the tones, her episodes became less frequent and less severe, her mood improved and she became capable of being on her own. Clearly, healing from the inside-out was happening for her. Thanks to Sharry, what Adrienne is experiencing in her recovery is a true miracle."

Cerebral Palsy

Just as a rainbow is incomplete without its full spectrum of colors, the body needs full-spectrum sounds that are created by the corresponding harmonic sets to establish and maintain the perfect state of health. The following case addresses both issues.

Young Owen's birth trauma left him with incurable cerebral palsy, a condition marked by impaired muscle coordination (spastic paralysis) and other disabilities. It is typically caused by damage to the brain before or at birth.

When I first met Owen, he was a cute two and half-year-old with an engaging smile and a loving personality, but he had no clear vocalizations. His parents were adoring and wanted only the very best for Owen. When they were told about my work, they quickly applied to be a part of the unique research using sound as a potential investigative tool for Wellness Providers.

Since the research I do depends on vocal biomarkers, it was a problem obtaining a vocal sample to be used for analysis of Owen, but Owen's father was determined that he was going to capture sounds from Owen that would provide the needed 30 seconds of a vocal print. Sounds of laughing, babbling, and gurgling were provided to my Institute, allowing Owen to be accepted as a research subject. Would Owen's "sounds" contain enough variety to create an accurate evaluation?

Although the Institute now uses computerized analysis to acquire bioinformation, the technique has esoteric beginnings: using "tones" produced by my voice to make the connections between sound and health. We occasionally revert to what we considered, in the past, to be an unsophisticated mode of gaining frequency-based information. For example, when there was a comatose or otherwise non-verbal subject to be evaluated.

Could this little-known, unique aspect of Sound Health's past protocols be useful for Owen's case study? I decided to find out.

When Owen arrived at the Sound Health Lab, our quickest solution was for me to "sing" his "Signature Sound" (see Chapter 2). Before beginning work with Owen, I verbalized a tone but laid the information aside for later scrutiny.

As the session progressed, Owen was soon verbally responding (more than cooing) to his grandmother, and we were able to get a full vocal print that provided us with the frequency ranges that we needed. Owen was fascinated and became very alert when we played back his own verbalizations.

The computer analysis indicated that Owen needed to be evaluated for stem cells, muscle proteins and nutrients, inflammation, metabolism, nerve recruitment/stabilization, and brain development. Only after we completed his evaluation and provided tones for him to take home, did I look back at the sounds I had verbally provided. Sure enough, three of the four sounds I sang to him were on his list of the 24 vocal frequencies that the computer chose for us to consider. The frequencies correlated to nerve sheathing, glucose metabolism, creatine, neuregulin (associated with myelin formation), and nebulin (associated with muscle integrity), plus several muscles for his feet, lower legs, and toes that we had just been working with. Owen's vocal print corroborated the toning I had provided. The sounds we provided for him to use at home confirmed that my ears and voice were indeed able to discern what he needed to support his energy body, which, I believe, is what arouses the physical body's healing potential.

Owen's case is only one of many instances of using my voice and ears to identify the Signature Sounds that all of us create and convey silently to others throughout our lives. I think this was a common occurrence for everyone long ago when sound was a part of our social interactions, and before lying became a part of our society and we began to doubt our own perceptions.

Hip and Joint Pain

Recent statistics from the U.S. Center for Disease Control and Prevention, report that nearly 70 million Americans suffer from chronic joint pain, stiffness, and inflammation.

Hip joint pain can run the gamut of being an intermittent annoyance, to causing relentless debilitating symptoms. Suggestions for relief can range from simple stretching movements and OTC pain relievers, to replacement of the entire hip joint and connective tissue with accompanying narcotics and corticosteroids. Surgery is often a last resort but still does not guarantee freedom from pain.

Causes of hip pain can be single or multiple in origin, including tendonitis, arthritis, bursitis (inflammation of joint fluid sacs), fibromyalgia, prolonged abnormal posture, osteonecrosis (restriction of the blood flow to the area), herniated discs, sciatica, trauma (due to repetitive or stressful movement, injury or excess weight), bacterial infection, and genetics. Inflammation commonly accompanies these symptoms but the cause of joint inflammation is not completely understood.

Stiffness, swelling, tenderness, fluid collection, lack of balance, instability, decreased mobility, and deterioration of bone and connective tissue often accompany joint pain. Often surgery and/or attempted rehabilitation is not completely helpful.

I conducted a small study to investigate the potential of pain relief and accompanying inflammation using vocal profiling and low frequency sound presentation. This option, if demonstrated to be viable, would offer non-invasive, easy-to-use, low-cost sound presentation as an option for pain reduction. Such a system would certainly be a welcomed resolution for people with chronic hip joint pain. However, it is not likely that such an efficacious alternative would be well-received by those whose financial status would be negatively impacted as a result of pain reduction without the use of prescribed pain medications and/or surgery.

It is generally recognized that joint pain stems from inflammation and that inflammation comes from either pathogenic or inflammatory mediators of the body. Although these are important issues when dealing with pain, this study primarily investigated the potential to identify and eliminate joint pain using Human BioAcoustic low frequency sound presentation.

Vocal sample data was used to develop appropriate formulations that were presented to each test subject during the testing phase of the process. All frequencies are reduced to appropriate octave levels and presented in the range of 0-64 Hertz, the frequency range required for brain wave entrainment. Objective biofeedback such as oxygen saturation, temperature, and heart-rate variability were monitored to determine optimal frequency-based combinations for each individual. Final tones chosen for use were set on a tone box (tone boxes are discussed later in this chapter) that delivered the appropriate formulations via headphones or an amplified subwoofer.

Case studies, to date, have shown that homogenous groups of people suffering from hip and other types of joint pain have strikingly similar needs in terms of frequency presentation and productive outcomes. This small sample study of three subjects, all of whom presented with active hip joint pain and associated symptoms, supports that premise.

Subject 1 was a 61-year-old male physician in general good health (he was a former jogger) with the exception of hip joint pain that had continued despite a myriad of contemporary and alternative treatments. He was contemplating joint replacement surgery in the immediate future, and reported constant right hip joint pain, stiffness with lack of balance and mobility of the joint and accompanying muscles. Walking was somewhat "jerky" with uneven steps. Muscle stiffness lessened with active movement. His pain level on the day of evaluation was estimated to be 5-6 on a scale of 1–10.

Subject 2 was a 30-year-old male graduate student who had undergone right hip ball- joint replacement surgery two years previously. Elevated cholesterol and depression from the constant pain and the lack of mobility was taking a toll on his energy and stamina. His joint stiffness lessened somewhat with movement, but his pain was obvious, and he suffered from a limp, which he described as a "hitch" that impaired his walking and balance. As part of his work, he was required to carry heavy equipment. This exacerbated his pain considerably, particularly when it was necessary for him to climb steps. His pain level on the day of evaluation was estimated to be 6–7 on a scale of 1–10.

Subject 3 was a 62-year-old female educator who had experienced a stroke two years prior. She also suffered from high blood pressure and diabetes and was taking five prescribed medications. A lack of weight management exacerbated her hip and joint pain, although her pain and stiffness was intermittent, and her muscle stiffness lessened with movement. She reported hesitation of movement at times, especially after periods of inactivity.

She could not correlate symptoms with any particular activity or possible allergy-causing foods. She also suffered from intermittent leg cramping at night. Her pain level on the day of evaluation was estimated to be a 3–4 on a scale of 1–10. Because her pain was intermittent, a comparison vocal sample was taken when pain was absent.

When considering appropriate formulations for each of these three subjects, brain dominance, the frequency of each Sonostat imaging (Sonostat is a form of ultrasound that uses high-frequency sound waves to produce images of veins in the body), and each subject's objective and subjective feedback was considered. Each frequency listing was developed independently and individually designed to identify and support the elimination of each subject's reported symptoms.

Among these three subjects, several nearly identical frequencies appeared in all three of their sets of vocal samples. A total of 192 Sonostat images from eight vocal samples were evaluated. Of these, 25 Sonostat sets matched the samples of at least two subjects, and seven sets matched all three subjects. The most diverse variance from the median was .06 hertz, a difference not discernible by the human ear.

Each set of appropriate tones was placed on a proprietary tone box that emitted analog duplicates of the sounds that were presented to each test subject during the testing phase of the process. One particular set of whole-brained frequencies eliminated the pain within minutes for all three subjects: For the physician, in less than one minute, he reported that the "results were impressive". Increased mobility and balance was reported by all three subjects, as well.

For Subject 2, his limp was reported by him, and observed by clinicians, to be less pervasive. There was a shift toward more fluidity in his gait. Stiffness was not eliminated but it was significantly diminished, and his walking was less hesitant.

The physician (Subject 1) was doing well, reporting that the pain had subsided until his tone box ceased working several days later. At that point, his pain returned after a day of not using the tone box. Because the pain seemed to go away so completely and seemingly effortlessly, he had

convinced himself that it was just time for the pain to fade. As a practic-
ing physician, he also reasoned that the elimination of pain could not be
as simple as listening to sound frequencies to have the pain subside. But
when the tone box quit working, he quickly realized the power of low
frequency sound presentation for the relief of hip joint pain.

Subject 2 required reassessment because one of the frequencies presented seemed to be causing headaches. A re-check of his vocal frequencies resulted in one of his tones being eliminated. Once this was done, his
headaches were no longer an issue with long-term use of the sounds in
his tone box.

The continued requirement for the sound frequencies long-term
is generally required to allow the joint structures that were damaged to
recover. Meanwhile, the probable biochemical root cause of the original
deterioration can also be addressed. Identifying Sonostats that decrease
the most apparent pain allows for the gathering of the most obviously
involved frequencies.

Because math can be used to compute predictable outcomes, the
missing Sonostats can be calculated. As a simple example: If we know that
$2+2+? = 10$, we can determine the missing component of the equation.
Known formats garnered from years of study allow us to consider absent
Sonostats which facilitate the construction of exacting sets of biofrequencies which can be used to ascertain the developing process and genetic
origins of presenting symptoms.

The following chart lists the seven consistent frequencies exhibited
by the test three subjects. In this chart the musical notes associated with
the frequency range of each Sonostat have been listed, with the common
frequency-based biomarkers used to diminish chronic hip pain for all
three subjects are shown in red.

Subjects	Note	Alleviated Pain	Frequency Equivalent™ Correlation		
Subj 3-NoPain	C		B12 co factor	sulfur pathway related	
Subject 2	C		tyrosine	muscles contain high levels of tyrosine	
Subject 3-Pain	C		Betacarotene	may help prevent formation of free radicals	
Subject 1	C		homocysteine	sulfur pathway related	
Subject 1	D		Myostatin Inhibitor	testosterone	DHEA
Subject 3-Pain	D		THF	5 methyl folate	may improve flexibility
Subject 2	D		tetrahydrofolate	AKA THF	THF active form of folate
Subj 3-NoPain	D		part of precursor pathway for methione and sulfur - required for collagen		
Subj 3-NoPain	D		Pycnogenol	activates production of collagen	
			related to antidote for arthritis bacteria		
Subject 1	D		Glutamine		
Subject 3-Pain	D		wheat sensitivity genome		
Subject 1	D		alpha keto glutarate		sulfur precursor
Subject 2	D		lysine		
Subj 3-NoPain	D#		NAD precursor	NAD free radical inflammation related	
Subject 1	D#		inflammation related		
Subject 2	D#		myelin protein		
Subject 2	D#		nerve sheathing related		
Subject 2	F		Vitamin C	essential for formation of collagen	
Subject 1	F		MTRR - part of 5 methyl folate pathway		
Subj 3-NoPain	F		B12 and homocysteine	related to sulfur pathway	
Subject 1	F		Methionine sulfoxide reductase	regulates antioxidative defenses	
Subject 2	F		hip muscle - Psoas major		
Subject 3-Pain	F		galactosamine		
Subject 2	F		glucosamine		helps supress inflammation
Subject 3-Pain	A		Ankle muscles		
Subject 1	A		Vitamin B5	potent antioxidant	may reduce joint pain
Subj 3-NoPain	A		lecithin		
Subject 1	A		manganese	enhances growth and repair bones	
Subject 2	A		phosphatidly choline		improves reflexes
Subject 2	A		required for repair and maintenace of myelin sheathing		

One particular set of notes (C in Subject 2, D in Subject 1, Subject 3-Pain, and Subject 2, and F in Subject 1 and Subject 2) eliminated the hip joint pain for all three subjects.

There are a great many frequency associations that relate to inflammation, including parts of the sulfur pathway (which is required to create collagen and connective tissue), evidence of free radical involvement which causes inflammation, ankle and hip muscles, plus assorted biochemicals relating to muscle health.

The results achieved by these three test subjects in this sample study demonstrate that hip joint pain elimination could be the starting point for establishing a standard process for pain relief using Human BioAcoustic vocal profiling and sound presentation. For the subjects in this study it was not necessary for them to know how the process worked, only that they had their life back, free from their relentless joint pain. In light of our current deteriorating health care system, a repeatable system capable of equivalent results as has been demonstrated by this small pilot study should not be viewed as an optional arena of exploration. It should be designated as mandatory.

Gout

Gout is a form of inflammatory arthritis that is caused by high levels of uric acid in bones, leading to the formation of sharp, needlelike crystals in the joints. It is characterized by sudden and severe pain, swelling, and redness in the joints, especially in the big toe and upper foot. But it can also strike other areas of the body, such as the lower back, ankles, knees, wrists, and fingers. It is often associated with a diet high in purines (found in red meat, shellfish, alcohol, and sugary drinks), hypertension, obesity, genetic mutations, kidney disease, other medical conditions, and certain medications.

Gout symptoms can be debilitating and persist for days at a time or longer, with flare-ups often recurring in people who are prone to develop gout. The incidence of gout flare-ups can be unpredictable, often occurring suddenly and without warning. Over time, recurring gout attacks can lead to chronic joint damage and other health complications. An estimated 12 million people in the US experience gout pain and flare-ups each year, with the incidence of gout attacks continuing to rise, especially among men in general, and among both older men and women.

Traditionally, gout is typically managed through dietary modifications and other lifestyle changes, along with medications, such as the drug colchicine, steroids, or nonsteroidal anti-inflammatory drugs (NSAIDs). The downside of such medications is that they can cause debilitating gastrointestinal side effects.

Human BioAcoustics and the vocal biomarkers it analyzes have emerged as a promising alternative to such drugs, leveraging voice analysis to diagnose and monitor health conditions. This innovative approach provides new insights into gout and offers alternative pathways of pain relief. Studies have associated uric acid with diabetic joint pain. Gout frequencies can usually relieve such pain.

Gout responds very well to Human BioAcoustics sessions. So much so, that I've developed a specific tone box called G-Out that people can order to prevent and relieve gout attacks. It's available at www.bioacousticsolutions.net/store, along with other tone boxes dedicated for preventing other specific health conditions.

An example of how rapidly Human BioAcoustics can resolve gout issues occurred years ago during a group class that I was teaching. At that time, Dr. Jonathan Murphy, MD, was participating in a BioAcoustic Vocal Profiling Training for medical professionals in which the class was evaluating the potential of pain relief using low-frequency sound. Being both skeptical and curious, Dr. Murphy inquired if there was a sound that would eliminate gout pain, which he was currently experiencing. His big toe often swelled, turned red and was very painful if he ingested certain foods or drink, especially when he imbibed whiskey, which caused the most pain for him.

The class and I decided to set up an experiment as a group intervention using the sound frequency combination that I had identified for pain relief. Dr. Murphy listened to the frequencies under headphones. Within a minute, the frequencies not only relieved the pain almost instantly but began to obviously decrease the redness and swelling in his affected toe and foot area. The event was recorded, and I've made the class video available to the public to show that Dr. Murphy was incredibly pleased that the sound frequencies successfully relieved his discomfort. You can watch the video at https://tinyurl.com/62mdvjr6 .

Vocal Biomarkers: A New Frontier In Gout Management: As I've explained throughout previous chapters of this book, vocal biomarkers have proven to be an innovative approach to health diagnostics because of how the analysis of voice patterns can reveal underlying health conditions. By analyzing the frequencies and patterns within a person's voice, it is possible to detect imbalances and identify potential health issues.

In the context of gout, vocal biomarkers provide a noninvasive method to monitor the condition. For example, changes in vocal frequencies might indicate an impending flare-up and provide other insights into the body's inflammatory state. This allows for early intervention, helping to prevent or mitigate the severity of gout attacks.

The Institute for BioAcoustic Biology & Sound Health has documented many cases of gout relief when gout sufferers listen to the specific low frequency sound frequencies that I've developed to treat gout. In the vast majority of cases, the relief of gout pain when the frequencies are listened to is often less than a minute, as the video of the above case history with Dr. Murphy shows.

The relationship between vocal biomarkers and gout lies in the body's biochemical processes. Gout is linked to metabolic disturbances, particularly the overproduction or under excretion of uric acid. These metabolic processes are reflected in the body's frequency patterns, which can be detected in the voice. By analyzing these patterns, vocal biomarker technology could potentially identify signs of metabolic imbalance before they manifest as a gout attack. For instance, specific frequency disruptions in the voice might correlate with elevated uric acid levels or inflammation. This information could be used to adjust treatment plans, dietary recommendations, or lifestyle changes to prevent flare-ups.

Moreover, vocal biomarkers can also be used to monitor the effectiveness of other gout treatments. By tracking changes in voice patterns over time, healthcare providers can gain insights into how well a client is responding to medication or other interventions. This could lead to more personalized and effective treatment strategies, reducing the frequency and severity of gout attacks.

Although gout remains a challenging condition to manage, with flare-ups causing significant pain and discomfort, Human BioAcoustics and Vocal Profile analysis of vocal biomarkers offers new, side-effect-free avenues for diagnosis and treatment. By leveraging the power of sound and voice, these innovative approaches could revolutionize the way we understand and manage gout, providing gout sufferers with more personalized, effective, and holistic care. As the science behind vocal biomarkers and sound therapy advances, we may one day see these techniques integrated into mainstream healthcare, offering a new standard of care for gout and other metabolic disorders. Until then, Human BioAcoustic sound therapy represents a promising area of exploration for those seeking alternative and complementary approaches to healing.

Macular Degeneration

Macular degeneration, also referred to as age-related macular degeneration or AMD, is a condition in which the macula, the part of the retina responsible for detailed and central vision, deteriorates, causing vision loss. It is one of the leading causes of vision loss among older adults, and is most common among older Americans, particularly white women over the age of 65, although it can occur earlier in life, as well. It is estimated that as many as 20 million Americans currently have AMD, with approximately 1.5 million of them afflicted with the vision-threatening late stage of AMD.

There are two types of macular degeneration: dry (non-neovascular), with dry macular degeneration being more commonly diagnosed, and making up 85 to 90 percent of all cases, and wet (neovascular), which may cause more profound vision loss, making up the remainder of cases. Dry AMD is caused either by the thinning of macular tissues or a deposit of drusen, or yellow spots, between the retinal pigment epithelium and the choroid beneath it. Those who suffer from early dry AMD may continue to have good vision for a while. However, as the condition progresses, it will cause gradual loss of central vision. The loss of vision for someone diagnosed with wet AMD, which dry may progress to, will typically become far more serious.

Conventional medical literature states that there is no cure for AMD. However, the following case studies support the reversal of macular degeneration using the low-frequency sound presentation techniques of Human BioAcoustics. The participants involved were all suffering vision loss due to macular degeneration. Their physicians had given them little hope, leaving them to search elsewhere for an alternative to their failing eyesight. This quest for a better prognosis and optimism brought them to my Research Institute.

Dorothy suffered from dry macular degeneration, and was not diagnosed until she was 82 years old. At that time, she had areas of her vision missing and was unable to even see her lip in the mirror because of the deterioration of the macula. She was distressed because she was not able to completely observe her sewing, nor could she see well enough to continue her church choir activities.

Upon her first visit to work with me, after commencing tone trials of the appropriate sounds indicated by her vocal print, in less than an hour, she was again able to see the "missing" part of her lip and through ongoing sessions she reversed the hole in her vision that once hindered her sight. Not only was her "blind spot" reversed, but several other factors, like brightness of the visual field, also improved. Dorothy has been undergoing tone trials for almost six years now, and her physician is pleased that her AMD has not only not progressed, but has improved.

Dorothy's Vocal Profile revealed that the Frequency Equivalent of the lens of her eye was below normal limits. In less than two minutes of low frequency sound presentation, Dorothy had no problem seeing herself in the mirror. Sounds were presented for an additional thirty minutes. Twelve hours later, with no sound frequencies, her vision was still intact. With continued Human BioAcoustic intervention, Dorothy's vision continues to remain stable.

Several additional study participants with AMD showed marked improvement following treatment with the sound frequencies their vocal profiles indicated they would benefit from, but Dorothy's case was one of the most noteworthy, possibly because her case was identified early.

Robert was diagnosed with wet macular degeneration when he was 64 years old. At this time, a lack of light caused his vision to be severely limited. He was unable to operate a vehicle at night due to his inability to perceive parked vehicles alongside streets. Road signs, even those with large letters, were unclear to him until he came directly upon them. It was also impossible for him to identify objects in a low light environment.

This inability also began to influence his work performance. Robert's job involved driving a cart in and out of a plant warehouse. The bright, natural light outside would temporarily—for a time span lasting up to 30 minutes—blind him upon re-entering the fluorescent lighting inside the plant. Furthermore, he suffered from a lack of depth perception, as objects commonly appeared closer than they actually were.

Robert's condition is most likely genetic, as his mother also suffered with AMD. Once his condition was identified, Robert's doctor not only told him that he was going to have to endure this condition for the remainder of his life, but that if he lived long enough, he would eventually go blind. Robert refused to accept this, but knew that something must be done. Having heard about my work, he decided to give it a try.

During his first visit, I performed an assessment of his vocal frequencies and began experimental tone trials. Two years after Robert completed his first Human BioAcoustics session and continued working with me, he regained all his vision except for a small hazy section. When he faithfully listens to his tones, he reports that he has the ability to see in a low light room. When asked how BioAcoustics makes him feel, he stated: "It's given me freedom."

Robert continues receiving regular Human BioAcoustic check-ups for readjustments as his eyes further progress towards full normal function. Conventional medical practitioners had repeatedly informed Robert that nothing could be done to improve his eyesight. Yet, there has been such dramatic improvement in his vision since he began using the Human BioAcoustic techniques I developed that Robert now only visits his medical practitioner to document his improvements.

Pauline was first diagnosed with dry macular degeneration when she was in her early sixties. Her condition can also be ascribed, at least in part to genetics, and she recalls memories of her mother, who would strategically place her grandchildren within her line of peripheral vision in an attempt to see their faces. Pauline admitted that she, too, had to take similar measures in the past.

According to Pauline, her optometrist was the first person to detect the granules in her eyes, though it took nearly seven years before the condition actually affected her vision. The way she described the transition from dry macular degeneration to wet is that a tiny spot is distorted in the affected eye and gradually grows to become a "blind spot". Her blind spot continued to grow until, three years later, it scope spanned the size of a quarter, which is visually the range of 17 characters on a page of print. Like Robert, she was also had problems seeing at a distance, and was completely unable to view remote colors.

Pauline travelled from Australia to see me since there were no methods of treatment available to her there. After about ten seconds of listening to the appropriate sound frequency, she could see a haze through the blind spot, though not clearly. After several days of listening to the frequency tones, she was able to see complete letters within the holes and eventually the span of her impairment decreased, as did holes in her vision. She even regained the ability to see rich colors myopically.

"It wasn't the first sound you tried," she told me. "Or the second or the third, so I was sitting here thinking, 'Nothing's happening.' But by the tenth sound, things began to improve. I wasn't expecting it, because you think nothing's happening and then suddenly the right sound, after listening to it for only ten seconds, enabled me to see letters and colors. It's amazing!"

Bleeding with Macular Degeneration: Mary Margaret suffered from macular degeneration and bleeding in her eye, both of which she was able to reverse once she began working with me and receiving the appropriate sound frequencies. Here, she relates her experience in her own words:

"One morning, the most remarkable thing happened. My left eye stopped bleeding! For the entire last year, I've had small bleeds on the upper right quadrant of my retina and a small bleed in the middle of the retina toward the bottom of my left eye.

"Since then I have stayed on the tones Sharry created for me, and my eyes are most definitely improving. More light is moving through the blind spot. In addition, more good news is that the special glasses I was prescribed by the Sight Center to wear are now too strong. However, nothing could have prepared me for what happened the following week. I went to a new ophthalmologist. After examining my eyes, he said he had to change my prescription for my contact lenses because my vision has improved. You may wonder why on earth I was wearing contact lenses. The lenses are to correct what little vision remains, my peripheral vision. This is the same prescription I had for probably 15 years, and at least eight years before the time I had gotten ill. Yet the doctor was now telling me that my prescription was too strong! This means not only is my peripheral vision expanding, and the vision I do have is sharper and I can discern color, and light is coming thru the blind spot, the non-blind part of my eyes are also improving. I thank Sharry for giving me back my song and with that song, my laughter."

Today, Mary Margaret is no longer legally blind. She doesn't use her glasses except to read. She can drive herself around and is in great spirits. Her sight is returning, she has returned to a full-time career, the macular degeneration has receded, and she is energetic and ecstatic about her new life.

Given the lack of options people with macular degeneration have, the research results that my staff and I have achieved have proven not only to be innovative, but necessary. Human BioAcoustics is the only noninvasive means of aiding the body in correcting issues thought to be incurable by conventional methods, including age-onset macular degeneration. This novel method of sound healing is turning heads and, literally, opening eyes (no pun intended) with its potential as a treatment for AMD.

Autism

Jocelyn was six years old when she began to work with me. She had been diagnosed with hypolexia, a form of autism, which had affected her since the age of three.

A Vocal Profile revealed that Jocelyn was likely highly sensitive to bovine protein found in cow's milk and other dairy products. Changing her diet has relieved the symptoms of autism. Even her ingestion of a small amount of milk can cause autistic symptoms to reoccur. Low-frequency sound presentation was able to relieve the symptoms should she accidentally ingest milk or milk protein.

Although the Human BioAcoustics technique used with Jocelyn is considered experimental, the discovery of the effects of bovine protein that analysis of Jocelyn's Vocal Profile revealed is consistent with other known causes of autism. Jocelyn was found to be sensitive to bovine milk from birth. If you compound this information with the fact that some vaccinations are cultured on milk and wheat proteins, it follows that the vaccination may have contributed to her allergic responses in that the symptoms started a few months after she received her standard MMR immunizations.

Infectious Diseases

Throughout history, humankind has been plagued by infectious diseases. With the advent of modern biochemical antibiotics, many of these diseases seem to have been eradicated. However, many new diseases have subsequently been identified, some of which are mutations of previously "cured" diseases in the form of drug-resistant pathogens. Our entire ecosystem has now become vulnerable to these drug-resistant pathogens due to the fact that, as these invaders move from host to host, they mutate so that what once worked against them may not work today. Antibiotic-resistant bacteria is a prime example of this, and has caused extreme concern for those in charge of public health. If we don't have the resources to keep up with the mutations, how can the public be protected? How will the people even know how to take precautions against infection?

Controversial researcher Hulda Clark, PhD, ND, stated in her book, *The Cure For All Disease*, that cancer, one of the most feared of diseases, is caused by pathogens, specifically, parasites whose life cycles are aided and abetted by modern chemicals that are so prevalent in our environment.

Clark is certainly not alone in identifying links between parasites/pathogens and modern illness. Chronic fatigue syndrome (CFS), for example, shows a strong connection with the Epstein Barr virus, and both heart disease and pulmonary embolism (blood clots in the lungs) have been connected with *Chlamydia pneumoniae*. The list of infectious agents and their link to various diseases is long and growing.

To add to this problem, these pathogens are able to use the body's processes against it. Using the sloughed-off protein of the host, they have the ability to create a protective cloak so that the body's immune system will be fooled into thinking that the pathogen is part of the body's normal form and function.

What can be done to combat this problem? For years, I have been conducting studies using Human BioAcoustics to help find answers. The Human BioAcoustics technology I've developed has been shown under microscopic observation to be able to dissolve the ringed protein barrier used by some of these pathogens to cloak themselves. The technique has been used successfully against the Epstein Barr virus, *Chlamydia pneumoniae* bacterium, and yeast, among other pathogens. It has potential in the eradication of such diseases as CFS, influenza, HIV/AIDS, etc., and it certainly helps in the fight against antibiotic-resistant pathogens including the resistant «flesh-eating bugs» which have been in the news.

At the beginning of my research in this area, the frequencies identified in Dr Clark's book were used, but I found that these were either not accurate or that mutations in the pathogens had taken place, thus making these frequencies unusable. This necessitated a search for new, correct frequencies.

What follows is a short review of the initial study I conducted, which involved 17 participants in which their infections of Epstein Barr virus, the *Chlamydia pneumoniae* bacterium, and/or yeast were targeted. (Note that in the case of the yeast, the decloaking and deactivation happened so quickly that the yeast could not be seen after a minute or so.)

Epstein Barr Virus (EBV): A filmed recording of the activity under the microscope shows that when the coating of the Epstein Barr virus was dissolved, the neutrophils (white blood cells that attack invaders) were activated. The activity of the neutrophils was nil until the EBV was decloaked by the appropriate sound frequency, even though the two were separated by minute distances. As the decloaking transpired, it was obvious that the neutrophils had not been aware of the EBV until the protein coating had begun to dissolve. After the decloaking, the neutrophils went to work to consume the invading pathogen.

Here are some additional notes from the study:

1. The sound frequency for dealing with EBV is listed by Dr Clark as having the musical note of C#, but I found it to range from mid C# to early D.
2. When the EBV pathogen numbers were high, there was an active invasion as well as corresponding symptoms (the most common being fatigue) which varied in intensity.
3. When the antigen sound frequencies were high, antibodies were being produced by the participants' immune system.
4. When detoxifying the Epstein Barr virus, ear and throat infections, pain and sensitivity in those areas were noticed. Reports show that Epstein Barr virus tends to hide in the neck area.

Chlamydia pneumoniae: Human BioAcoustic voice spectral analysis has been shown to be an inexpensive and quick way to determine which pathogens are present and which antibodies have been manufactured by the body. In the case of Chlamydia pneumoniae, I was able to identify those participants in the study who had been infected by the bacterium, those who had created antibodies to it, and those who were on their way to being free of the infection.

Additional notes from the study are as follows:

1. This bacterium was not listed by Dr Clark.
2. This is not the sexually transmitted variety of Chlamydia; the *Chlamydia pneumoniae* strain is airborne and it attacks the lungs and pulmonary system. Its symptoms include labored breathing, dizziness and passing out, accelerated heart rate, high blood pressure and muddled thinking. Re-infection is possible after symptoms have disappeared. The bacterium has an incubation period of 10-14 days.
3. The frequency of *Chlamydia pneumoniae* corresponds with the musical note of C#, and also involves the note of A, which is associated with blood clotting.
4. For active cases, a narrow band of C# was active in each chart, and late A to early A# was also involved.
5. For those with high protease levels, symptoms did not appear. (Protease is an enzyme that digests proteins.)
6. For those with blood type O, symptoms were short and less severe.
7. When the Frequency Equivalent of Chlamydia was high, an active infection was present.
8. When the antigen sound frequencies were high, antibodies were being produced.
9. The *Chlamydia pneumoniae* formed clots which formed a protective coating that cloaked the entire clot from the neutrophils. These clots are not shown in chest X-rays or clotting factor scans. It is suggested that a pulmonary arteriography or a spiral CT of the lung be ordered to verify the presence of these small clots in the lung tissue.
10. Eating fatty foods or heavy meals exacerbated symptoms of labored breathing. Depending on how much fatty food or how

large the meal had been consumed by the participant, symptoms would dissipate within half an hour to four hours after treatment. Participants who had poor digestion of protein were most vulnerable. A high dose of the enzyme protease was used along with digestive enzymes to ease or dissipate the symptoms.

11. Doxycycl HYC, a potent antibiotic, is reported to be able to kill this strain of *Chlamydia pneumoniae*, but had little effect in this case. Giving the Frequency Equivalent for Doxycycl produced side effects as if the medication had been given, even though the subject had never taken it before.

12. One infected, particularly vulnerable client exhibited small, thin, pinch-like bruises.

13. One client had a pacemaker implanted by doctors to stop an accelerated heart rate, but the breathing problems and muddled thinking were still present after the placement of the pacemaker.

14. One client was told that he needed heart surgery to clear blocked arteries, but, obtaining a second opinion, he discovered that this was not necessary.

15. One client, despite being infected before the start of the study, was told by the medical establishment that absolutely nothing was wrong, except simply stress.

Before becoming participants of the study, four persons in the study ended up in the hospital, but not one hospital discovered that a pathogen was causing the problem.

The above study confirmed that voice frequencies can identify pathogens and also provide mathematical frequency sets that can assist the body eradicate them. This was further demonstrated in the following case history.

Laura was extremely tired. Her medical tests provided little help, although a blood examination using a darkfield microscope confirmed that Laura had Epstein Barr virus. The frequencies of Epstein Barr also show up as an invading pathogen in her vocal print. A mathematical set of formulas was developed and used to decloak the pathogen and assist her body to identify the intruder. Once the pathogen was decloaked, the natural killer (NK) cells of Laura's immune system easily identified and attacked the EBV The sound frequencies Laura received not only worked well to eliminate the EBV, but also the pathogenic bacteria and yeast in Laura's body. Because of her Human BioAcoustics treatment, she was able to soon resume her active lifestyle.

COVID-19

In December 2019, the Institute of BioAcoustic Biology & Sound Health published the frequencies associated with the frequency-based antidotes for COVID-19 based on my research.

I had been following naturally occurring flu cases for more than a decade and determined that the math platform of COVID-19 did not mathematically match any long-standing, naturally occurring viruses. I noticed a change in the mathematical patterns of COVID-19 compared to other viral pathogens. The numbers were too perfect. They did not match Nature's viral and other pathogen matrixes. The genes and protein antidotes were in conflict with each other, and we concluded that these frequency combinations were man-made. Nature-made pathogens have antidotes that are not harmonic. These current COVID-19 virus frequency antidotes are numerically harmonic. This indicated to me that COVID-19 was likely man-made. It took nearly two years for that information to be publicly scrutinized, and it is now commonly accepted by most scientists that COVID-19 was indeed bioengineered by humans.

Along with issues of fatigue related to iron and glucose usage, the published COVID-19 frequencies mathematically included vitamin D, quercetin, glutathione, nitric oxide, platelet aggregating factors, and zinc, likely leading to the probability that vascular issues were going to become prevalent. Autopsies consequently presented by pathology professionals substantiated that these frequency-based calculations were correct. Subsequent studies published in multiple medical journals have now shown that both COVID-19 and the mRNA vaccines, both of which include a novel spike protein, are causing an increase in the incidence of myocarditis, pericarditis, and other related heart conditions.

Some of the frequencies of COVID-19 are also associated with HIV. The data compiled by the Institute of BioAcoustic Biology & Sound Health showed that the virus would cause respiratory difficulty, severe fatigue, stem cell damage, blood clotting, inflammation, and circulatory issues. Everything my colleagues and I reported then has now been investigated and reported in medical journals and by the mainstream media.

Then, in 2023, we discovered an additional COVID-19 variant, Pirole (aka BA 2.86), being forced upon an uncertain public. It has taken many dedicated people to decode the variants associated with Pirole. Mathematically speaking, these frequencies, to our horror, are primarily associated with infertility and miscarriage, cases of both of which have sky-rocketed following the pandemic and the mass mRNA vaccination agenda.

I have developed a free service that anyone can use to determine if they are still unknowingly being affected by COVID-19. To use it, go to SoundHealthPortal.com/coronaconflicts, choose Covid 23 as your template, and then leave a vocal sample. Results comparing your vocal frequencies to Covid 23, will be emailed to you. Remember to use an appropriate microphone, or your results may not be accurate. Follow the directions found on the Portal. If these frequencies are in your vocal report, go to your trusted wellness provider for advice.

Le Ciel: In the Introduction to this book, you read about how Human BioAcoustics was responsible for actor James Marshall's complete recovery from a life-threatening gastrointestinal condition. My computerized analysis of his voice indicated which nutrients James needed in order for his body to heal itself, as well as which foods would support his healing, and which foods he needed to avoid. I also provided him with the sound frequencies that would help him heal.

"I started using this information and my life began to fall back in place," James reports. "My mind began to clear, I started to gain weight, and my energy returned." Eventually, James completely regained his health by using the sound frequencies and following the dietary and nutritional recommendations his Vocal Profile analysis determined that he needed.

"I started playing the frequencies on my guitar," James says. "It was not the same as playing music; it had a greater impact on me. I spent hours with the sounds and I began to feel like my old self."

Since his recovery, James and his wife have worked with me to study Human BioAcoustics and sound healing. Eventually, they came to me *wanting to focus on the work I'd done with the swine flu virus. I decoded the genetic make-up of the strains of swine flu and their* frequency biomarkers, and was able to mathematically determine the frequency based antidotes, which I shared with James, who began putting them to music. In the process, he created a sound recording called Le Ciel, which seems to influence and reverse symptoms that are pathogenic in nature.

"I discovered that this would not sound like a traditional song," James explains. "I had to remind myself it would be a musical piece meant to kill a pathogen in the body. *It became the musical piece called* Le Ciel *and has shown signs of doing just that. My wife, myself, and others have found relief from cold and sore throat symptoms. In addition, the frequencies have been used to reverse swine flu symptoms that were resistant to Tamiflu."*

You can download an eight-minute version of LeCiel for free at soundhealthoptions.com/product/le-ciel-8-minute-version-2 or purchase the full 18-minute version at soundhealthoptions.com/product/le-ciel-18-minute-version-2/.

Note: Please know that neither James nor I make medical claims about LeCiel. It is available for research purposes only.

Voice Frequencies Can Identify Biochemical Toxins

One summer, seven-year-old Andi, previously a top reader in her school class, had forgotten how to read. Her teacher demanded that Andi be put in a special reading class. This embarrassed Andi and made her reluctant to go to school. She cried every day. On the days she didn't cry, she pretended to be sick.

Her parents brought Andi to be evaluated by Human BioAcoustics technology. Vocal testing was used to determine if there were any biochemical reasons for Andi's reading problems. During that session, while she was receiving low-frequency sound, Andi was able to read clearly and without hesitation. The test pointed to the possibility that Andi had been poisoned by formaldehyde, a chemical preservative.

A detoxification program was initiated, and Andi's teacher noticed immediate and striking differences in the girl. Andi's self-esteem soared. She was again a bright, cheerful, intelligent child. Best of all, she could read again!

World Trade Center Toxins: Two Human BioAcoustic group studies were conducted for personnel working at the World Trade Center (WTC) devastation site caused by the terrorist attacks on 9/11. The first study showed the consistent toxins found within the vocal prints of the engineering personnel working at Ground Zero. From this study, a potential cause of the Fireman's Cough was determined and later confirmed for a small sample of volunteers.

A second study done at the invitation of the Fireman's Union confirmed the findings of the initial study. An in-depth evaluation of the data revealed that an early age onset breast cancer gene has an identical frequency as the toxin that seems to be causing the Fireman's Cough.

My Sound Health Institute was invited to evaluate the hundreds of additional personnel working at Ground Zero. Funding is the only obstacle that kept this research from moving forward to include everyone that may have been affected by the WTC toxins.

BioAcoustic Vocal Profiles Depicting Toxin Frequency Equivalents for Persons Working Near WTC after 9/11: The prevalence of 13 specific toxin Frequency Equivalents that were identified from the vocal prints of eight engineering personnel working at Ground Zero.

3 of 8 subjects – Bromochloracetic Acid

5 of 8 subjects – Hexane

3 of 8 subjects – Styrene-D

5 of 8 subjects – Methacrylic Acid

3 of 8 subjects – Acrolein

5 of 8 subjects – Bromine

5 of 8 subjects – Benzoflouranthene

3 of 8 subjects – Potassium Cyanide

5 of 8 subjects – Vinyl Acetate

4 of 8 subjects – Silver Aluminum

5 of 8 subjects – Mirex

5 of 8 subjects – Sodium Cyanide

5 of 8 subjects – Phthalic Anhydride.

The ability of Human BioAcoustics technology to detect these toxins demonstrates its effectiveness and potential as a toxin screening tool for the general public.

Voice Frequencies Can Ascertain Muscle Stress, Trauma, And Weakness

Bob was an attorney and a motorcycle enthusiast. Five years before he came to work with me, Bob had an accident that was so severe that the doctors wanted to amputate his leg. Being an avid tennis player, Bob refused to allow the operation, but he did undergo several major surgeries, with additional reconstructive surgery to create the illusion that his leg muscles were intact. Bob's physicians had little hope for a complete recovery and told him to consider himself lucky to be alive. After two years of physical therapy there was little hope that he would ever be able to walk normally again. The lowest section of his leg was as large as a football. He could not walk straight nor bend his ankle, and his stamina for any exercise was gone. Bob closed his law practice and went home to his parents who lived in a small community in Ohio. He felt that his life, as he wanted it to be, was over.

One day, while he was grocery shopping, Bob met a fellow tennis player, who told him about my Research Institute and that I was conducting experiments to test the idea that low frequency sound could be used to help recover muscle strength and control. For Bob, the idea of using sound to heal seemed a far-fetched notion. "I'm a lawyer and an engineer, so I was skeptical," he said, but he had little to lose and nothing else had helped, so he dubiously decided to give it a try.

Bob met with me and his voice was analyzed. A portable tone box was then programmed to emit the sound frequencies analysis of his vocal print indicated might help him. Bob was very intrigued by the obvious effect that the sounds from the tone box had on his muscles, which became apparent soon after he began listening to the sound frequencies.

Today, Bob is no longer a skeptic about my work. "The swelling is gone," Bob reports. "There is no pain anymore. I don't even think of my leg as being injured anymore. I had severe limping and couldn't run at all. Now I can run, dodge, and jump. I'm now matching Bill [the person he met at the grocery store] on the tennis courts step for step, which is something I never thought I would be able to do."

The sound frequency program I designed for Bob worked specifically with the muscles of his lower leg to help the body stimulate muscle tone and pain relief. Both Bob and I were surprised that he improved so dramatically, to the point that he now gives tennis lessons and plays tennis whenever his busy schedule allows.

Two months after working with Human BioAcoustics, Bob was back on the tennis court giving the locals a challenging workout. He could walk straight; he could almost run; he could chase a tennis ball. The swelling dissipated and his leg now had muscle tone and movement. He had his life back again and he was ecstatic. Bob was doing so well on the court that he was asked to be the tennis coach at the local high school.

In another case, a female jogger was referred to my clinic because one of her legs was two inches shorter than the other one due to the trauma of a hit-and-run incident. An operation was scheduled to try to elongate the bone.

Analysis of her voice print was able to show that a thigh muscle was very tight. Low-frequency analog sound was presented to relax the muscle. Within a few minutes of muscle manipulation, both legs were the same length, and, with exercise, have continued to remain in the normalized state, sparing her of the need for the operation.

Other Case History Examples

The following cases histories were documented by Liz Lonergan, RN. Liz is a certified practitioner of Human BioAcoustics and treated each of the following clients using the sound healing diagnostic and treatment methods I've developed.

Bladder Weakness and Incontinence: A woman named Mary Lou came to Liz suffering from bladder weakness, a chronic urgency to urinate, and incontinence. She was a very active senior who was troubled by this 'inconvenience,' as she termed her condition. Previous to seeing Liz, she chose to forego any medications for her issue, and always needed to be close to a bathroom or wear a sanitary pad, which was taxing on her confidence as a teacher of yoga and Qiqong classes.

Human BioAcoustic Evaluation conducted by Liz revealed Frequency Equivalents for two perineal muscles that assist in bladder control that were identified in her vocal print. The appropriate frequencies tested positively for Mary Lou, and her bladder problem was under control within a week. "All I can say is thank you," she told Liz. "I have my confidence back, and that is priceless."

Knee Injury: James was a senior in college. While playing football, he took a nasty hit from the side. Medical reports revealed that he had incurred torn medial and lateral collateral ligaments, a torn posterior cruciate ligament, a torn medial meniscus, and a medial femoral condyle fracture of his left knee. When he came to Liz, his left knee was swollen, he was in a lot of pain, and was unable to bear weight on or bend his knee.

His doctors told James that he would have to have two surgeries, and at least one full year of intensive rehabilitation to regain the use of his knee. His football career was over and he would probably have to put his college career on hold for a year as well. His fiancé had heard of Human BioAcoustic analysis and suggested he try it before making any decision on surgery. He was two weeks post-injury when he came to Liz for evaluation, wearing a locking full leg brace and on crutches.

Several vocal samples from James were taken over two days. They revealed Frequency Equivalents for inflammation in many of the muscles that have attachments on the medial side of the knee. During tone trials, James' brace was unlocked for his comfort. To his surprise, James was able to move his knee on his own while listening to the sound frequencies Liz prepared for him. (He was unable to move his leg without assistance before the sounds). The muscles and tone frequencies that James responded to the best were put on a tone box and he returned home.

James listened to the sounds faithfully for 1.5 to 2 hours a day. At the end of four weeks he was pain-free, his knee and leg were again weight bearing, and had regained 50 percent of the range of motion. By the end of three months, James had regained 99 percent use of his knee. Within six months, he had finished his college studies without interruption, and had resumed his martial arts and yoga practices.

"I was skeptical at first, but my doctors and I are positively startled by the speed and completeness of my recovery," James stated. "I would definitely recommend this therapy for everyone."

Thumb Pain Combined With Thyroid Imbalance: Arianne came to Liz suffering from a thumb injury and severe depression. She had a loss of range of motion in her thumb and fifth finger, and was also experiencing hair loss and low levels of energy. She was a massage therapist and regaining the full use of her hand was her main priority. She had refused antidepressant medication suggested by her doctor and was treating her thumb injury with self-massage.

However, Arianna's Human BioAcoustic evaluation indicated Frequency Equivalents for the potential of thyroid issues, which included stress involved in her body's utilization of thyroid hormone and iodine. The Frequency Equivalents suggested she might also have trouble utilizing serotonin, an important brain chemical that gives one a sense of wellbeing.

Her voice test also showed Frequency Equivalents indicting a potential difficulty using collagen, which is necessary for tissue repair, along with several thumb and hand muscle imbalances.

Based on these findings, Liz prepared specific sound frequencies for Arianna to listen to. After the first night of listening to her tones Arrianna stated, "I felt as though a dark, heavy weight had been lifted from my chest. I felt great!" She continued listening to her tones and took some suggested food supplements Liz recommended. Within two weeks, she had regained full range of motion in her thumb, showed no further symptoms of depression or thyroid imbalance, and her hair had stopped falling out.

"I am so glad that we are finally reaching the technological advancements to offer this kind of gentle, non-invasive healing therapy to people," Arianna says. "Surely this will benefit humankind far more than I can even appreciate."

Presumed Multiple Sclerosis (MS): Lisa came to Liz reporting generalized muscle weakness, especially in the legs, and low energy levels. After being thoroughly evaluated by her doctors, Lisa was found to have all the clinical signs of MS, including lesions on her brain and spinal cord. Her doctors had tried all the conventional MS drug protocols with her, but she had been unresponsive to treatment.

When she was evaluated by Liz, her vocal analysis repeatedly showed Frequency Equivalents in infection architecture, with an Frequency Equivalent for herpes simplex virus 6 (HSV6). During Human BioAcoustic tone trials, Lisa responded positively to the Frequency Equivalent of Acyclovir, a drug commonly used for treating viral infections. Liz referred back to her MD and she tested positive for the HSV6 virus.

When Lisa returned to continue with the Human Bioacoustic testing, she was placed on tones for fighting the virus and supporting her body. After six months, she was reevaluated by her doctors and was found to be free of the lesions found previously on her brain and spinal cord, and she had no more symptoms of MS. Today, Lisa enjoys an active life and has resumed her career in teaching.

"This is the most amazing thing I have ever experienced," Lisa says. "If it weren't for Bioacoustics, I would still be suffering and being treated for the wrong illness. I have been given my life back!"

These case histories not only illustrate the effectiveness of Human BioAcoustics, but also demonstrate how anyone, with proper training through my Research Institute (see Chapter 9), can achieve these same type of results to provide hope and healing in their community.

Dedicated Tone Boxes

Before concluding this chapter, I want to provide a brief overview of the dedicated tone boxes I've developed for managing specific health conditions and related issues, such as the G-Out tone box I discussed above.

The following dedicated tone boxes that are available to the public.

G-Out™ Dedicated Tone Box: Gout is characterized as one of the most painful forms of arthritis that presents itself in the form of severe pain, redness, and tenderness in the joints, most often in the big toe. The G-Out™ dedicated tone box is designed to help reduce the strain and symptoms of gout.

Front to Back™ Dedicated Tone Box: The Front to Back™ dedicated tone box works on core energy and back muscles while you sleep. It focuses on balancing and maintaining the muscles in your core and back. Back muscles give power to the body, playing a major role in all the body's functions. They connect the hips, butt, chest, shoulder and neck. Among other uses, this tone box is perfect for women who are pregnant.

Face Time Continuum™ **Dedicated Tone Box:** Wrinkles are a natural part of aging, and are most prominent on sun-exposed skin, such as the face, neck, hands, and forearms. Skin structure is predominantly determined by skin texture. However, sun exposure is a major cause of wrinkles, especially for people with light skin.

Apart from the natural aging process, other major factors can cause wrinkles, such as smoking, poor nutrition, dehydration, and feeling stressed or tired.

The Face Time Continuum™ dedicated tone box addresses facial wrinkles and loss of tone due to the ravages of time, free radicals, and aging.

BioBody™ **Dedicated Tone Box:** Physical activity can cause muscles to become fatigued, sore and inflamed. The BioBody™ dedicated tone box contains the frequencies necessary to help your muscles recover from activity while you sleep. The frequencies travel through your muscles, stimulating and relaxing them with sound. BioBody™ balances all the muscle components in your body with the designated sound frequencies to ensure they remain strong and healthy.

Fab Abs™ **Dedicated Tone Box:** Abdominal muscles support the torso, allow movement, and hold organs in place by managing internal abdominal strain. They encircle and support the spine and pelvis, while connecting a person's upper and lower body, essentially transferring forces from one to the other. A strong core also leads to better balance and stability, whether you are performing daily activities or engaging in vigorous physical exercise. The Fab Abs™ dedicated tone box is designed to work on core energy and abdominal muscles while you sleep.

Muscle Factors™ **Dedicated Tone Box:** Muscles produce lactic acid during intense exercise as a metabolic byproduct that leads to muscle fatigue and soreness. Relieving it can help the nutrients in your body create more energy, relieve sore muscles, and prevent muscle cramps. This Muscle Factors™ dedicated tone box helps the body clear lactic acid.

It is perfect for athletes or individuals who engage in frequent physical exercise and contains the frequencies necessary to help individuals who endure the symptoms of fibromyalgia.

The frequencies in the tone box are able to remove unwanted chemicals and minerals, such as iron excess, that are stored in your body. An iron overload may disturb the delicate balance between bone resorption (the process where the body absorbs cells or tissue, often involving the breakdown of structures like bone) and bone reformation, which can weaken the bone. This Muscle Factors™ tone box can help with musculoskeletal pain and other symptoms caused by fibromyalgia.

Little Black Box Dedicated Tone Box™: Pain experts and economists agree that back pain is the most frequent cause of activity limitation and lost work hours. The Little Back Box™ was designed to provide temporary relief of back stress, but it was not designed for long-term trauma or pain. It is expected that your use of the Little Back Box will be over several sessions, each providing longer and more sustained relief.

Overture™ Dedicated Tone Box: This dedicated tone box tunes up basic DNA/RNA frequencies. DNA and RNA are two different types of nucleic acids that are crucial for cell functioning, and therefore, for life.

Both DNA and RNA carry genetic material, but there are many differences between the two. DNA is the blueprint for life as it contains all the genetic material in a cell that will be passed down when reproduction occurs. RNA provides the codes for amino acids so that when they are transported to ribosomes in the cell they can form proteins crucial to maintain the cell's functioning.

The Overture™ dedicated tone box contains the frequencies to help tune up basic DNA/RNA frequencies and keep them strong and healthy.

Pumping Iron™ Dedicated Tone Box: Whether it be 5G or COVID-19 pandemic residue, bioacoustically speaking, both situations have been found to be closely involved with the use of iron within the body. Not just the presence of iron but with its use via iron regulatory proteins. Research completed in December 2019 confirmed that iron regulatory proteins have a direct mathematical relationship with the gene and proteins associated with the pandemic. This dedicated tone box support iron regulation and utilization in the body.

Radical Relief™ **Dedicated Tone Box:** When the atomic bombs that fell on Fukushima and Hiroshima were detonated, vast numbers of people in the nearby vicinity were greatly affected by radiation poisoning. Radiation breaks down and weakens DNA, and can damage cells enough to kill them or cause them to mutate in ways that can cause people to contract fatal diseases like cancer. The Radical Relief™ tone box uses frequencies to help people recover from damage to the body caused by radiation.

Restless Legs™ **Dedicated Tone Box:** Restless legs syndrome is the feeling in the legs that there is too much energy and they need to move or jerk. Serious issues with restless legs feel like you are being hit with a stun gun or cattle prod. The Restless Legs™ dedicated tone box is designed to calm the muscles in your legs so you may be able to work and sleep painlessly.

Charlie Chaser™ **Dedicated Tone Box:** Charlie horse muscle cramps can occur in any muscle at any time, but they can be prevented. They can be from inadequate blood flow to the muscles, excessive hot or cold weather, dehydration, and not stretching/being mindful of your body during exercise. These cramps are most likely to occur in athletes, older adults, and people who are taking medications like diuretics or statin drugs. The Charlie Chaser™ dedicated tone box will help eliminate the stress of Charlie horse and other muscle cramps using specific frequencies.

Teeth Integrity™ **Dedicated Tone Box:** Dental pain is one of the most common forms of pain people experience. This pain can be caused by tooth decay, tooth abscesses and fracturing, as well as infected gums and other issues that arise from a lack of dental hygiene. Tooth pain can be related to almost anything in the body, including issues with the nerves, enamel and pulp channel that make up a healthy tooth. The Teeth Integrity™ dedicated tone box uses frequencies to support dental health by keeping the nerve, enamel, and pulp channel that surround the teeth healthy and strong.

Pythagoras Series™ Dedicated Tone Box: Pythagoras is credited with creating the first documented musical tuning system based on 432 Hz as the note of A. He calculated mathematical ratios using string. This dedicated tone box provides his frequency-based system combined with the sound frequencies for human chakras.

Myalis™ Dedicated Tone Box: This tone box emulates the effects of cialis medication to dilate blood vessels, lower blood pressure, and increase sexual ability in both male and female users.

Note: Unlike on customized tone boxes that use the specific frequencies that are based on the findings of an individual's Vocal Print, the frequencies of dedicated are preprogrammed and should work for anyone seeking to use them. Each purchase includes a pair of Koss headphones for comfortable listening to the frequencies.

To purchase a dedicated tone box, visit www.bioacousticsolutions. net/store.

Conclusion

These examples of healing that I've shared in this chapter represent only a small fraction of the information that can be gleaned from vocal prints. The successful treatment outcomes I've shared above cover only a small list of conditions for which Human BioAcoustics can help. In addition to viewing the body as a mathematical matrix, Human BioAcoustics considers the idea that frequencies can be used to predict states of disease and

BREAKING THE SOUND BARRIER OF DISEASE

stress before they become obvious on a physical level. Protocols are being developed to identify the frequency relationships for cancer, heart disease, arthritis and sports injuries, regeneration and antiaging. The study of numerous vocal prints permits researchers to recognize obvious frequency markers for various states of illness.

The field of Human BioAcoustics, utilizing the idea that frequencies contained in the voice are holographic representations of one's state of health, were it to be more widely adopted and used, could significantly improve health outcomes safely, quickly, and inexpensively.

Research has repeatedly shown that every muscle, compound, process, and structure of the body has a Frequency Equivalent that can be mathematically calculated. This provides the foundation for the concept that the body's ability to heal itself can originate as frequency interactions between the molecular signals of the entire body. When these patterns become discordant, *dis-ease* is the result. When presented with the correct low-frequency analog sound, a new harmony can result, with the person experiencing notable self-healing.

CHAPTER 6

HUMAN BIOACOUSTIC THERAPY AND WEIGHT MANAGEMENT

I t's no secret that, as a nation, unhealthy weight gain and obesity pose serious health risks for many Americans. According to the Centers for Disease Control and Prevention (CDC), obesity currently affects four out of 10 Americans. Even more alarming, the trend towards unhealthy weight gain and obesity is now affecting children, pre-teens, and teenagers at greater levels than ever before. The CDC reports that 12.7 percent of two- to five-year-olds, 20.7 percent of six- to 11-year-olds and 22.2 percent of 12- to 19-year-olds in the U.S. today are obese. Obesity is a primary cause of many chronic medical conditions, including type 2 diabetes, some forms of cancer, heart disease, osteoarthritis, and gallbladder disease. In addition, medical costs for people with obesity in the U.S. tend to be 30 to 40 percent higher than those for people who aren't obese.

It is a common misconception that eating less and increasing exercise is the panacea for weight loss. This is far from the truth. In this chapter, I am going to reveal to you how and why Human BioAcoustic therapy can effectively help people who are overweight shed unwanted pounds and keep them off. You will also discover other important steps you can take to get your weight under control and become healthier.

What Vocal Profile Samples Reveal About Unhealthy Weight Gain

A survey of people who volunteered their vocal prints indicated that the most insidious stress for them was body image and their inability to manage weight loss successfully. Why does weight loss seem to be so individual, so elusive for them, and for overweight people in general?

Bioacoustically speaking, people with similar issues have similar vocal frequencies. Based on that tenet, the Sound Health research team and I attempted to answer this complicated question.

Over 2000 vocal prints of volunteers were evaluated. Twenty generalized categories were found. One very obvious but elusive culprit was revealed. (See #20 below).

Many people reported that they failed so often to lose weight that they just wanted to give up.

What follow are the categories that we found to be at issue for them based on a Human BioAcoustics analysis of their vocal prints.

1. **Thermogenesis**: Thermogenesis refers to the production of heat in the body, contributing to energy expenditure and weight loss. Increasing thermogenesis is one method for promoting weight loss, as it can raise the number of calories burned even at rest.

Ingesting heat-producing foods can increase thermogenesis. Green tea, capsicum (cayenne), chili peppers, and caffeine can also trigger thermogenesis. Caffeine also increases adrenaline. (**Note:** I generally do not recommend caffeine as, for many people, it can act as an unhealthy, addictive drug.) Extracts of Garcinia cambogia, a tropical fruit, are often used in weight loss supplements because of its thermogenetic effects.

The body is very redundant. Almost every frequency has many correlates of muscles and biochemistry. The jaw muscles of chewing (e.g., the pterygoid and the masseter together) create the frequency of dopamine, a biochemical associated with satiation. Thermogenesis issues are often associated with the thyroid. A vocal print analysis can detect such issues, and can also evaluate your balance of white and brown fat that manages excess adipose tissue.

2. **Medications:** Many medications, including weight loss drugs, can be toxic and contribute to weight gain. Certain ones, like some antidepressants, steroids, and anti-psychotics, can lead to weight gain as a side effect. Prednisone is also known for its ability to cause weight gain.

A new class of drugs called glucagon-like peptide-1 (GLP-1) receptor agonists has become the latest craze in weight loss medications. GLP-1 is a gut hormone that regulates blood sugar and appetite. These drugs were originally developed to help manage symptoms of type 2 diabetes, but soon became used by physicians to address unhealthy weight gain and obesity with or without diabetes. They mimic GLP-1, and include Ozempic, the most popular drug in this class. A similar class of drugs mimics both GLP-1 and GIP, another gut hormone receptor. Mounjaro is one of the most popular drugs in this class, and was specifically developed to help with weight loss. However, both classes of drugs have reported many negative side effects, and I do not recommend them.

3. **Neurotransmitters:** Neurotransmitters, released from the brain, interact with other neurotransmitter receptors.

Neurotransmitters such as serotonin influence sleep; GABA, glutamate, acetylcholine, dopamine, and serotonin are involved. Serotonin signaling is involved in eating behavior regulation and long-term body weight. These and other weight loss biochemicals and hormones are included in the Ultimate Diet template you can access on the free public WorkStation my team and I developed at SoundHealthPortal.com.

4. **Biochemistry:** Leptin, AMPK, adiponectin, alpha lipoic acid, and berberine are just a few of the weight management biochemicals included in the BioDiet template on the Portal that you can use to assess Human BioAcoustic frequencies associated with weight management.

5. **Medical Conditions:** Polycystic ovary syndrome (PCOS), certain endocrine disorders, diabetes, menopause, fatty liver disease, and genetic conditions can increase the likelihood of obesity by interfering with body chemistry. These conditions can be evaluated by using the Human BioAcoustics Disorders, Hormones and Receptors, Leaky Gut, or Fatty Liver templates at SoundHealthPortal.com.

6. **Aging:** As people age, they often lose muscle mass, slowing their metabolism and increasing the risk of weight gain. This template is also in the weight management BioBundle on the Portal.

7. **Genetics:** A person's genes can significantly influence weight gain by affecting factors such as appetite, metabolism, and how the body stores fat. However, both lifestyle choices and environmental factors also play crucial roles and influence genetic predispositions for good or bad.

8. **Insulin Resistance:** One of the key pathways through which chronic inflammation contributes to weight gain is induced insulin resistance. Inflammation disrupts the normal signaling and function of insulin, a hormone responsible for regulating blood sugar levels. This disruption leads to higher glucose levels in the bloodstream and encourages fat accumulation in the liver. The presence of these conditions can contribute to weight gain and metabolic dysfunction.

9. **Thyroid:** Thyroid function is associated with energy production. Impaired or low thyroid function (hypothyroidism) is very common today. Fatigue is the most reported complaint. The Krebs cycle and thyroid templates on the Portal can help map methylation and cellular energy issues.

10. **Diabetes:** Taking insulin causes weight gain. Insulin is a hormone that regulates how the body absorbs sugar, also known as glucose.

For many diabetics, stomach weight gain can be frustrating. Diabetics also complain of adipose tissue gain on the lower side of the upper arm. The frequency of this muscle corresponds to an obesity gene. Insulin allows sugar to enter your cells, which decreases sugar levels in your blood. But if you take in more calories than are needed to keep a healthy weight, your cells will get more sugar than they need. This happens in people who do not have diabetes, too. How many calories you need depends on how active you are. Sugar that your cells cannot use becomes fat.

11. **Nutrition:** The body needs hydration, sunshine, minerals, vitamins, quality protein, and essential fatty acids in balance for the glands to produce the necessary hormones needed to function normally. When nutrients are deficient, the glands add extra fat and fluid as a backup defense mechanism to produce vital hormones. Once the glands are nourished and repaired, the fat will decrease.

Ghrelin and leptin are associated with appetite management. Both can be BioAcoustically evaluated using the BioDiet template.

12. **Insomnia:** "It's not so much that if you sleep, you will lose weight, but if you are sleep-deprived, meaning that you are not getting enough minutes of sleep or good quality sleep, your metabolism will not function properly," explains Michael Breus, PhD, author of *Beauty Sleep* and the clinical director of the sleep division for Arrowhead Health in Glendale, Arizona.

13. **Inflammation:** Markers that promote inflammation, such as IL-6, tumor necrosis factor (TNF), C-reactive proteins (CRP), and adiponectin, are closely connected to gaining weight. Factors such as stress, insufficient sleep, and consuming processed foods also play a role in fostering chronic inflammation and weight gain.

14. **Stress:** Research shows chronic stress disrupts immune function and can lead to inflammation. It can increase the risk of stress-related diseases due to mild chronic inflammation. Stress may also contribute

to weight gain, as the hormone cortisol is known to do. Managing stress is crucial for overall health and inflammation reduction.

15. **Hormones:** Hormones are important substances that serve as chemical messengers supporting optimal body maintenance. These include cortisol, insulin, leptin, ghrelin, estrogen, neuropeptide Y, GLP-1, cholecystokinin, and peptide YY (decreases appetite), all of which are included in the Weight Management templates at the Portal. Polycystic ovary disease and endometriosis are two of many hormonal weight-gaining disorders. The template to monitor these hormones is Hormones and Receptors.

16. **Peptides:** Various peptides, including human growth hormone (HGH), can be individually evaluated using the Weight Management BioBundle.

17. **Sarcopenia (Age-Related Skeletal Muscle Loss):** Intramuscular fat, like visceral fat, releases harmful inflammatory molecules and significantly affects muscle quality. Unlike subcutaneous fat (fat stored under the skin) or visceral fat (fat stored around organs), intramuscular fat infiltrates muscle fibers, thus degrading their performance and functionality. It can accumulate between muscle fibers or within muscle cells, causing weight loss and frailty.

A 2022 study in *Physiology Reports* showed that higher levels of intramuscular fat elevated inflammatory cytokines, contributing to metabolic disorders. The journal *Radiology* revealed that fat accumulation in skeletal muscles can increase the risk of death as much as Type 2 diabetes and smoking. The research, which tracked nearly 9,000 healthy adults over nine years, found that higher intramuscular fat significantly raises health risks. Exercise can dramatically slow the rate of muscle loss.

18. **Stem Cells:** Obesity has become a global epidemic and a threat to human health worldwide. It can be seen as an excess accumulation of adipose associated with heart disease, hypertension, inflammation, and diabetes. Templates to BioAcoustically evaluate stem cell status are part of the Weight Management BioBundle offered to the public.

19. **Inflammatory Cytokines:** Intramuscular fat releases pro-inflammatory cytokines, creating whole-body inflammation. Additionally, carbohydrates and processed foods contribute to intramuscular fat.

20. **Toxicity:** Above all other factors, an abundance of toxins and free radicals (found in pesticides, food additives, medications, body care and cleaning products, and animal growth hormones) are the number one commonality for people reporting weight management difficulties.

Fat cells store toxins that the body cannot process and eliminate. When you lose fat cells, those substances are released into the metabolic system, dumping lipids (fats) and environmental pollutants into the bloodstream.

One of the most common toxins today is glyphosate. Glyphosate is an insidious environmental pollutant. It has the same frequency as MSG, B12, and several B vitamin co-factors. Glyphosate could interfere with cellular energy, mood, detoxification of lymph and glymph systems, and lipids at a cellular level.

Not all fat is bad. In fact, fat is necessary for energy storage, insulation, organ cushioning, hormonal regulation, nutrient absorption, and brain/nerve health. Having healthy body fat is essential for optimal body form and function. Managing your fat is vital for good health. The wrong type or excess fat is detrimental, and too little healthy fat is equally harmful. Knowing what is causing fat imbalances could help support weight loss and optimally balance your metabolism.

Fat Hormones and Human BioAcoustics

When working with people who are struggling to lose weight, we use layers of sound frequencies to outline how layers of redundant frequencies create a physical map of why a person may gain weight. Basically, it's just the use of frequency layers to reveal each person's intrinsic mathematical constitution.

Musical octaves are the doubling or halving layers of mechanical vibration. For instance, the musical note of "A" is recognized as 440 hertz (cycles per second of mechanical vibration). A tuning fork vibrating at 440 cycles per second will create the musical note of "A." Half of that rate, 220 cycles per second of vibration, will create the note of "A" but at one octave lower.

Likewise, 110 cycles per second will produce a musical note of "A" at yet a lower layer. We live in a world of musical layers of octaves. Our body is built on these mechanical layers and responds to different octaves of frequencies, as color, sound, brain waves, nerve impulses, etc.

Our body operates within several layers of frequencies. Each system within the body produces a range of them and responds optimally to its precise octave and then favorably to the associated frequency of stress. For instance, frequencies for the eye are 60-90 cycles per second. Therefore, frequencies used for eye repair should be found within that range, with lesser supporting frequencies at multiples of the original frequency. Using this supposition, let's evaluate a few fat-burning hormones having frequencies akin to other body systems that may cause interference.

Layers of frequencies can be interpreted as layers of sound. Listed below are some fat hormones associated with weight issues. I hope you will be able to recognize system associations that can help identify your health issues. All these biochemicals have frequency equivalents. They are also in the weight management database at the Portal for comparisons using your vocal frequencies.

1. **Adiponectin:** BioAcoustically speaking, if this is low, you will likely experience eye focus and bladder issues. Among its functions, it increases the breakdown of fatty acids, and enhances insulin sensitivity. Higher levels are associated with lower body fat.

Adiponectin is one of the majorly distorted frequencies caused by Spike proteins.

2. **Glucagon:** BioAcoustically speaking, when glucagon is lacking, you may experience TMJ issues. Glucagon stimulates the liver to break down glycogen into glucose, and promotes fat breakdown (lipolysis) when glucose levels are low.

3. **Epinephrine (Adrenaline):** Human BioAcoustics testing shows that if this hormone is not balanced, you may experience thyroid issues. It activates fat breakdown by stimulating lipolysis, and increases energy output during stress or exercise.

4. **Norepinephrine:** When norepinephrine is low, my research shows that kidney energy may be unbalanced combined with vitamin B6 being low. Norepinephrine works alongside epinephrine to trigger fat breakdown. It is released during exercise and fasting.

5. **Thyroid Hormones, T3 and T4:** When these thyroid hormones are low, fatigue may be high, and use of iron low, accompanied by pain in the neck region. T3 and T4 regulate metabolism and energy use, and help mobilize stored fats for energy.

6. **Testosterone :** BioAcoustically speaking, when testosterone is low, you may experience muscle weakness, finger pain, and a lack of visual focus. Testosterone supports muscle growth, which increases resting metabolic rate. It also promotes fat loss, particularly abdominal fat.

7. **Growth Hormone (GH):** When GH is lacking, stomach muscle tone is weak, and accompanied by muscle soreness. GH stimulates the breakdown of fat. It increases during sleep, fasting, and intense exercise.

8. **Insulin-Like Growth Factor-1 (IGF-1):** BioAcoustically speaking, when IGF-1 is lacking, blood sugar may be unbalanced, and oxygen use by the body is insufficient. IGF-1 works in conjunction with growth hormones, and plays a role in reducing fat mass and increasing muscle mass.

9. **Cortisol (In Controlled Amounts):** Cortisol is known as the stress hormone because it is secreted by the body during times of stress. Chronically high levels of cortisol that persist throughout the day

can cause both inflammation and excess weight gain via fat storage, particularly in the abdomen. Balanced, or controlled, levels of cortisol mobilize stored fats during fasting or intense exercise. BioAcoustically speaking, however, low cortisol levels are often associated with upper back pain.

10. **Leptin:** BioAcoustically speaking, when leptin is lacking, lung surface proteins may be stressed. Leptin regulates appetite and energy. High leptin sensitivity encourages fat burning, while leptin resistance, like insulin resistance, can lead to fat accumulation.

11. **Irisin:** BioAcoustically speaking, when irisin is lacking, you may experience a low tolerance to temperature changes. Irisin is produced during exercise. It converts white fat into brown fat, which burns calories to produce heat.

12. **Peptide YY3-36 (PYY3-36):** Peptide YY3-36 is a protein hormone that is primarily secreted by the cells lining the small intestine in response to food intake. It plays a crucial role in regulating appetite and satiety by signaling the brain to reduce food intake and increase feelings of fullness. PYY3-36 acts on specific receptors in the hypothalamus, reducing appetite and promotes fat utilization, leading to decreased hunger and increased energy expenditure. BioAcoustically speaking, when PYY3-36 levels are low, you may experience joint pain and less flexibility.

In addition to these fat hormones, the amino acid carnitine is essential for fat burning. BioAcoustically speaking, if it is low, you may experience more food sensitivities.

Vocal profiling can help determine imbalances and deficiencies of these hormones, as well as carnitine, and sound frequencies specific to each individual based on their vocal print analysis can help optimize their levels in conjunction with balanced nutrition, regular physical activity, adequate sleep, and stress management, to improve fat-burning efficiency and enhance your ability to lose weight and keep it off.

Examples of Vocal Profile Findings

All of the associated frequencies relevant to weight loss have numeric equivalents that are included in the weight management database you can use on the Sound Health Portal. They are available for comparisons using your own vocal frequencies. (You can find instructions for how to do this at https://tinyurl.com/45rsav4f).

During one of my public presentations, hundreds of people visited our Sound Health Public WorkStation and volunteered voice samples to be evaluated. What follow are three examples that illustrate the capability of frequencies to identify potential weight management issues.

The Weight Management summary provides BioAcoustic generalizations from a myriad of diet related databases. Any percentage score over 2.0 percent reveals information of significant concern.

1. Martin's vocal print analysis found that his Lipid Liabilities score was 3.7, likely indicating a fatty liver that is either not producing or distributing the enzymes needed for digestion. A low fat diet is generally not the solution for correcting this. A gentle liver cleanse may be indicated since the liver produces and manages these biochemicals. Milk thistle or turmeric might also help Martin. A deeper evaluation may need to include cholesterol and co-factor scans.

2. Tonya complained of a lot of pain and upset in her digestion system from top to bottom. Her doctor blamed a lack of appropriate enzymes and severely restricted her diet. She stated that she could not budge her belly fat. A deep evaluation of her leaky gut symptoms showed the presence of an unnatural bacteria in her gut, as well as a severely disturbed gut lining, and a fatty liver that was not providing appropriate fat dissolving bile salts.

The digestive enzyme lipase helped relieve the major carbohydrate digestion stress Tonya was experiencing. Tonya also started to use Dr. Steven Gundry's gut lining restoration products with success.

3. TJ complained of a cranky digestion system and belly fat. He reported heart disease and a family history of vascular stress. His evaluation pointed to two issues: fatty liver and a leaky gut. A leaky gut indicates a loss of the mucous lining of the gut, causing bowel contents to leak into the abdominal cavity. This is generally a result of environmental toxicity by pesticides.

Dr. Gundry has the best products I've found for a leaky gut. Gundry also advises abstaining from lectin containing foods, such as beans, tree nuts, tomatoes, and peppers.

Muscle Frequencies As They Related To Weight Management

One of the main reasons why potential weight management issues can be revealed using frequency-based vocal analysis is because, as I am fond of saying, BioAcoustically speaking, almost everything is something else. Meaning that one frequency may, and often does, have many correlations. Body systems are redundant and interconnected and have many ways to reveal intrinsic secrets. Weight management issues can be analyzed visually using a map of where fat tissue tends to gather in the body.

The map below depicts muscle frequencies as they relate to weight management. By examining the location of fat molecules in the body the explanation for excess fat tissue be identified.

Muscle-Fat Storage Map

Lysine –
Fat burning peptides, fat storage
AMPK enzyme
Lungs
Liver
Adiponectin
Dopamine receptor
Bile use, Lipase
Taurine –
Insulin resistance
Adrenal stress
Lipase
Arginine –
Small intestine
Pancreas/ vitamin D
Thermogenesis
Adrenal stress and ATP conversion
Allergies
Adrenal

Being overweight is a massive problem in the US in nearly 60 percent of the population, leaving many people without a reasonable explanation of why they are overweight and can't slim down. For example, in another case history, Rachel, a 66-year-old with uncontrolled diabetes, high bad cholesterol, and high blood pressure, had been subjected to continued scolding, lectures, and new medications each time she visited her conventional medical provider. When her vocal print was evaluated using our online weight management template, her vocal analysis revealed the root cause of her weight issues to be inadequate lipid management.

Further questioning revealed that her gallbladder had been removed over 30 years ago, without any instruction given her to explain what would happen without bile salts to help break down fats. She continued to have gallbladder pain symptoms but modified her diet to avoid gastric issues.

The underlying cause was an inability to process lipids (fats), a concept not readily addressed by conventional medicine. Vocal analysis quickly ascertained that the issues were a lack of adiponectin and leptin. Adiponectin is the same frequency as the bicep muscle underneath the upper arm. This "bat wing" image is often associated with a physical manifestation of diabetes. (Adiponectin is a protein hormone involved in regulating glucose levels and fatty acid breakdown. In humans, it is encoded by the ADIPOQ gene and produced primarily in adipose tissue, but also in muscle and even in the brain.)

Rachel revealed she was very concerned about the hanging fat bags below her upper arms. The map of fat storage biochemical and muscle correlations above accurately depicted the biochemicals associated with her weight issues. Additionally, several bile salts, which are necessary to break down fat for digestion, were involved. Adiponectin and leptin were added to her supplement regime. The frequencies of both compounds were also provided to her via an analog tone box which entrains brain frequencies for use by the body. Since working with me, Rachel has reported more energy, better sleep, and feeling stronger and more flexible since starting this innovative protocol.

When incoming foodstuff comes into the body, your metabolism has two choices. Use it for energy or store it. The lack of adiponectin causes the body to store incoming calories, resulting in fat deposits.

Another person with whom I worked was Peggy, who needed help to find the root cause of her allergies and chronic rhinitis (a stuffed-up, drippy nose). Peggy had never found a health care practitioner who could provide a solution that would eliminate her symptoms. Her vocal print revealed a leaky gut, inflammation, and a fatty liver causing hormonal and metabolic symptoms. The offending allergens were caused by her leaky gut, but her gut issues were causing additional issues because of the inflammatory response it was causing.

Peggy was also experiencing unrelenting fatigue and blood sugar challenges. In addition, her thyroid was stressed. Her vocal analysis revealed a fatty liver from cholesterol issues, which turned out, BioAcoustically, to be genetic. This, in turn, was causing liver-related hormonal issues. She had been on statins for a while, but they made her so ill that she stopped taking them. She reported that her weight continued to climb, especially in her midsection.

Peggy reported so many seemingly unrelated issues that her health-care provider did not take her seriously.

Vocal analysis revealed issues with her body's energy cycle (Krebs cycle). She was not using the incoming resources that allowed her body to convert foods into fuel.

The frequencies of the oblique muscle near the waist are the same as biochemical frequencies that deal with thyroid and adrenal issues. Calcium usage can be stressful when a spare tire begins to accumulate around your middle.

The midsection of Peggy's body was accumulating fat as a part of the body's protection system against toxins. When a toxin enters the system, the body wants to eliminate the culprit, but if that is not possible at the time, the body will encase the toxin in a cocoon of fat and store it away to deal with later. A belly full of fat is indicative of a body full of toxins. To avoid any toxicity issues, I advise people to research how to detoxify toxins before starting a diet.

BioAcoustically speaking, it is not just one frequency that is involved in using sounds as body support, but the combinations of frequencies that can cause change. Breaking the code of obesity down to the root cause seems to still be a mystery for conventional medicine. Learning these combinations is what I teach and share with the public.

As an example, when adiponectin and leptin are combined, they influence the gracilis muscle so that as you walk, one foot is pointing to the side rather than straight forward.

Other concepts of muscle and fat tissue placement that have been borne out using vocal analysis include AMPK, lymph issues, pancreas, gallbladder, ghrelin, insulin resistance, and glymph system.

I invite everyone to check out a personalized Weight Management assessment at SoundHealthPortal.com. Also keep in mind that the amino acids taurine, lysine, and arginine are needed to produce bile salts necessary to break down carbohydrates and fats. These primarily relate to the throat and thigh muscles.

If you are interested in learning this protocol to share with your family, friends, and community, please check out our class information at www.bioacousticsolutions.net/portal-class-info.

Biochemical Causes Of Fat Storage In the Body

For many people, concentrating on how much food they eat, and how much exercise they do, is the essence of most weight loss programs. A lot of time and money is being spent on how to look good. The latest Ozempic, Mounjaro, and other weight-loss peptides craze is a good example of this. The outdated idea of eat less, exercise more is leaving those with unmanaged weight issues without hope or help.

Earlier in this chapter, I listed the most prevalent weight loss commonalities that have been shared with us. Without a doubt, toxicity was the number one culprit, followed by a fatty liver causing insulin resistance. Exploring this topic led me to the realization that fat tissue lays down and accumulates on the part of the body that has the most compatible frequency associated with the toxin or biochemical.

A lot of pesticide toxins accumulate in adipose tissue found on the frontal stomach muscles. Fat deposits are also often found on the lower side of the upper arms, and are said to be a diabetic body marker. That particular muscle (bicep femoris) has the same frequency as adiponectin. Adiponectin is involved in regulating glucose levels and fatty acid breakdown.

For more about where the body stores fat, see the fat storage map above. I created it in hopes of helping people identify the biochemicals associated with their individual weight loss issues.

Most people are not familiar with weight storage biochemicals. Organs such as the liver, gallbladder, pancreas, and intestines are involved. Even saliva produced when we chew food is involved in digestion. Many people who have had their gallbladder removed are never told that the gallbladder and liver are involved with the creation of bile salts which help emulsify incoming fats.

Taurocholate, a bile salt, along with amino acid taurine, aids in bile production and helps to emulsify dietary fat. Tauroursodeoxycholic acid (TUDCA) is a naturally occurring water-soluble bile acid. Bacteria in your large intestine break down bile salts and turn them into ursodeoxycholic acid (UDCA). UDCA then combines with taurine molecules to create TUDCA.

TUDCA has been used as a supplement for thousands of years in traditional Chinese medicine. It was first sourced from bear bile, which is made up of 50 percent TUDCA. Today, this health-promoting supplement is made synthetically.

As I mentioned, the body does two things with incoming foodstuff: It is used for energy or it is stored. Issues begin when energy is not created for immediate use but is stored and not readily available. Hence one of the first weight management issues to arise is fatigue. Fatigue is often associated with thyroid issues, a lack of fat burning, and slow metabolism. Cholesterol issues may be involved, as well.

In order for the body to properly and efficiently break down and digest (metabolize) food, it requires an adequate supply of enzymes and other biochemicals, as shown in this illustration.

→ FAT BREAKDOWN & ENERGY UTILIZATION ENZYMES
Fat-burning enzymes play a key role in breaking down stored fat into usable energy.

SOUND HEALTH
www.BioAcousticSolutions.net
1 (740) 698-9119

CATEGORY		ENZYME/PROTEIN	FUNCTION
Lipase Family (Breaks Down Fat)	→	Hormone-Sensitive Lipase (HSL)	Mobilizes stored fat by breaking down triglycerides into free fatty acids.
		Adipose Triglyceride Lipase (ATGL)	The first enzyme to act on triglycerides, converting them into diglycerides and releasing fatty acids.
		Lipoprotein Lipase (LPL)	Helps break down fats from the bloodstream so they can be used for energy.
Carnitine-Related Enzymes (Transport Fat for Energy)	→	Carnitine Palmitoyltransferase I (CPT1)	Moves fatty acids into mitochondria for energy production
		Carnitine Palmitoyltransferase II (CPT2)	Completes the transfer process for fat oxidation inside the mitochondria.
Beta-Oxidation Enzymes (Burn Fat for Energy)	→	Acyl-CoA Dehydrogenase	The first step in breaking down fatty acids inside mitochondria
		Enoyl-CoA Hydratase	Helps further break down fatty acids into smaller units for energy.
AMP-Activated Protein Kinase (AMPK)	→	Regulates Fat Burning	Not an enzyme itself, but AMPK activates fat-burning pathways by increasing energy expenditure and breaking down stored fat.
Boosting fat-burning enzymes naturally involves: diet, exercise, and lifestyle habits.	(How) →	Increase Protein Intake	·Protein stimulates hormone-sensitive lipase (HSL) and lipoprotein lipase (LPL), which help break down stored fat. ·Good sources: Eggs, lean meats, fish, nuts, and dairy.

Other fat-burning biochemicals include:

1. Peptides: Short chain amino acids involved in biochemical functions such as hormones, insulin and oxytocin.

2. AMPK: An enzyme that helps regulate energy balance in the body. It also manages cholesterol and fatty acid metabolism.

3. Taurine: A sulfur-containing amino acid important in the metabolism of fats and bile salts.

4. Lysine: An amino acid that helps build protein, collagen, bile salts and carnitine.

5. Lipase: An enzyme that helps digest fats. It is produced hormonally, and by the liver, pancreas, and salivary glands. Lipase is especially lacking in post-menopausal females.

6. Arginine: An amino acid that helps the body build proteins such as bile salts. It is found in many foods, including meat, fish, poultry, soy, beans, and dairy.

7. Adiponectin: A protein hormone that helps with insulin sensitivity, inflammation, and metabolic processes, especially with regard to fat cells released into the bloodstream.
8. Leptin: A hormone primarily produced by adipose (fat) tissue that plays a crucial role in regulating energy balance by inhibiting hunger, thereby helping to regulate body weight.

Efficient fat-burning also relies on your body's ability to produce ATP (adenosine triphosphate). This process releases energy that cells use to power their many functions. It involves energy conversion and expenditures at the cellular level, within mitochondria, the cells' "energy factories".

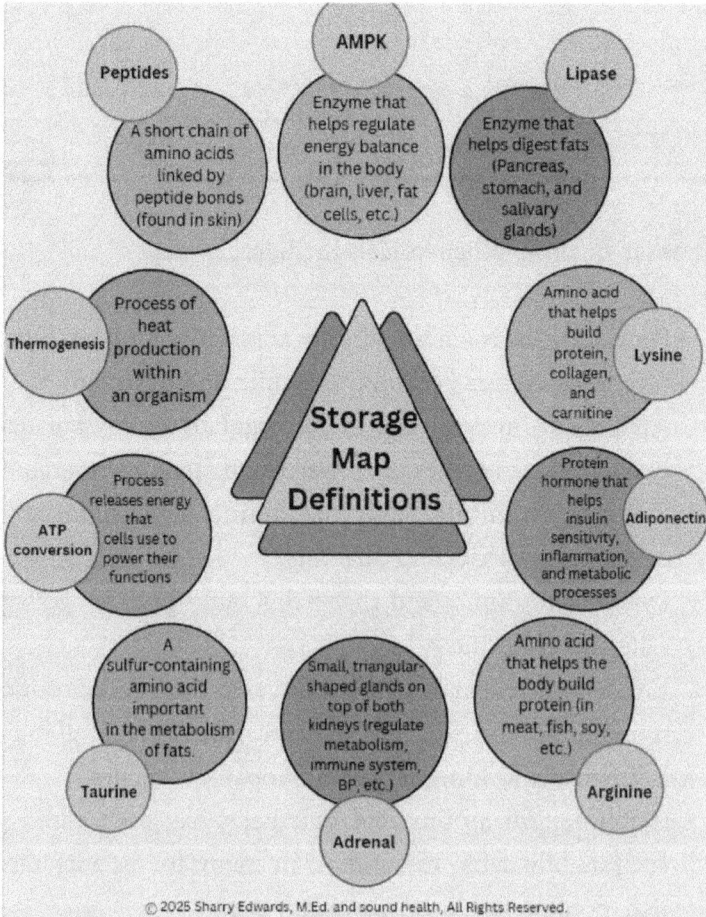

How A Sound Health Vocal Analysis Can Help

The most asked question I receive from our people struggling with weight issues has been how they can get a Human BioAcoustic online weight management evaluation. Once again, the quick solution is to go to SoundHealthPortal.com. Follow the prompts on the landing page that will lead you through the process, including inputting your vocal print. Within 24 to 48 hours, you will receive a preliminary report via email that will include a personal, computerized, quantifying report of your own vocal BioMarker anomalies.

What follows is an example of what's included in the report.

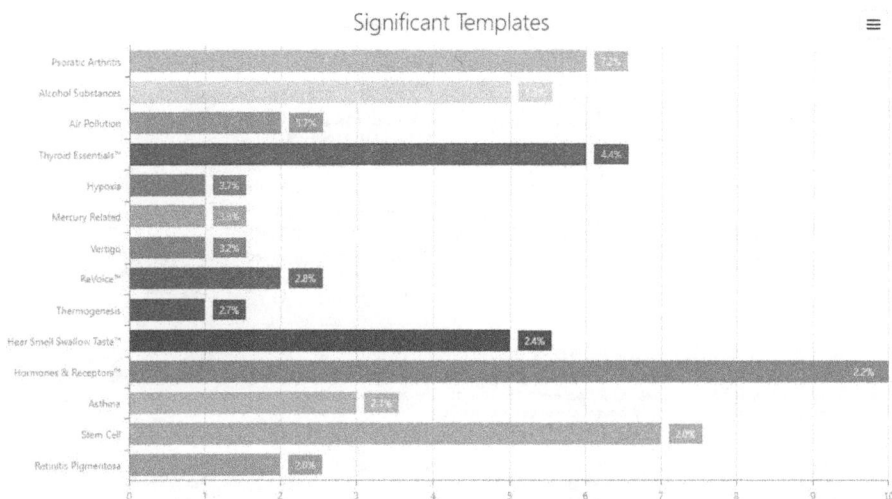

Significant Templates

This report, in particular, among other factors, identifies thyroid and thermogenesis as potential issues. Having cold hands and feet or trouble staying warm are usually noticeable symptoms. People with low thyroid function may need help from their health care provider to address that issue.

During my studies of the top 20 weight management issues, I found that one of the most often reported problems was a lack of information about past gallbladder stress. Few people were told what to expect or what could likely occur.

Using the Portal, a subsequent report with a gallbladder template may look like this:

Name: **Christina Client**				Rank
Research Results				Rank
Actigall	Medication	H	Used to dissolve gallstones; aka Ursosan	1
Chenodeoxycholic acid	Biochemical	H	Produced by the liver from cholesterol; 1 of the 3 major biliary bile acids	1
Cholesterol 7 Alpha-Hydroxylase	Epigenetic	H	Suppresses enzymes in bile acid synthesis	1
Sucrose	Biochemical	L	Excessive consumption may increase the risk of gallstones	1
Ursodeoxycholic acid	Biochemical	H	Bile acid produced by the liver and stored in the gall bladder	1
Ursodeoxycholic acid	Biochemical	H	May dissolve (cholesterol) gallstones; also known as Ursodiol	1
Ursodeoxycholic acid	Biochemical	H	Reduces the rate at which the intestine absorbs cholesterol	1
T-12 Thoracic vertebrae	Muscle - spine	H	Innervates gallbladder	2
Cynarin	Polyphenol	H	Chemical constituent of artichoke; may increase the flow of bile	3
Taurocholic acid	Biochemical	H	AKA: Cholaic Acid; a bile acid	3
Taurocholic acid	Biochemical	H	Constituent of bile; involved in the emulsification of fats	3
Acetyl Carnitine	Biochemical	H	Improves liver function	4
Cholic acid	Biochemical	H	1 of the 3 major biliary bile acids; produced by liver from cholesterol	4
Curcumin	Food Additive	H	May help prevent gallstones	4
Betaine Hydrochloride	Medication	L	Alkaloid that may reduce the risk of gallstones	5

In bioacoustic analysis, one of the challenges is that each detected frequency can correspond to multiple causes. This means that a single anomalous frequency might be linked to various factors or conditions, making it difficult to pinpoint the exact source without further analysis. This complexity requires careful interpretation to avoid misleading conclusions and to accurately identify the underlying issues.

The above gallbladder evaluation indicates if an item is High or Low and shows its priority on a scale of 1 through 5 that may need attention. The computer does the analysis for each individual. Each item has a blue line beneath it that is designed, when clicked, to take you to a resource. These reports can be shared with your wellness provider for potential remediation.

These protocols use information showing that the frequencies of the voice are a holographic representation of the body. Human BioAcoustic Biology has gathered information which indicates that the voice can potentially be used as a diagnostic tool but could provide sound-based solutions for health, including weight issues.

The online Portal includes tutorials, evaluations, documentaries, campaigns, articles, and references, plus the opportunity to scan your own voice for errant frequencies (sour notes). Record your voice and receive a personal report of what your voice reveals about you. And remember:

Your body is designed to heal itself. Sound-based frequencies can help it do so.

A Major Key to Stubborn Weight Loss

Non-alcoholic fatty liver disease (NAFLD) is a major key to stubborn weight loss. It is closely linked to weight management because it is both a cause and a consequence (effect) of metabolic imbalances tied to excess body weight.

A fatty liver impairs the functioning of digestive enzymes, the breakdown of fatty acids, the creation of bile salts, and metabolic hormone and biochemistry metabolism. It also exacerbates toxicity, insulin resistance, and chronic inflammation. For this reason, repairing your fatty liver may need to be your first step to effectively lose weight.

Fatty liver occurs when excess fat builds up in liver cells, impairing liver function. There are two types of fatty liver disease: AFLD (alcohol-related fatty liver disease), which is caused by excessive alcohol consumption and especially alcoholism, and NAFLD, which is not caused by alcohol, but is strongly tied to obesity and metabolic syndrome. NAFLD is typically caused by sugars and carbohydrates being turned into alcohol by the body. Common microorganisms implicated in this process include Saccharomyces cerevisiae, Candida albicans, and Klebsiella pneumoniae.

Fatty liver and weight are connected in the following ways:

1. **Excess Weight Increases Liver Fat.** When this happens, visceral fat (fat stored around organs) releases inflammatory chemicals and free fatty acids that end up in the liver. The liver then begins to store more fat, leading to NAFLD.

2.   **Insulin Resistance and Metabolic Syndrome.** Both of these conditions are common in overweight individuals. They can cause liver cells to take in more fat and produce more glucose, leading to a vicious cycle: more fat → more insulin resistance → fatter.

3.   **Fatty Liver Makes Weight Loss Harder.** A fatty liver can disrupt hormone signaling, as well as adiponectin, AMPK, leptin, fatty co-factors, and insulin, all of which make it harder to regulate appetite and energy production and energy use.

4.   **Weight Loss Improves Fatty Liver.** Losing just 5 to 10 percent of body weight can significantly reduce liver fat, improve liver enzyme levels, and reduce inflammation. Low-carbohydrate diets (Paleo, Ketogenic, or Carnivore) work for many people trying to lose weight. Going vegetarian may work for others. (**Note:** No single type of diet is suitable for everyone, and obtaining vital nutrients is necessary.)

Refraining from refined or artificial sugars (e.g., diet sodas) also greatly helps to reduce weight. Refined sugar spikes insulin and artificial sugar confuses the body's insulin responses even more. Refined carbohydrates do the same.

Some people use intermittent fasting to correct fat metabolism. This involves eating all of your meals in an 8 to 12 hour window each day.

Some people have had success using turmeric for weight loss, as well, because of turmeric's proven ability to improve liver function and reduce chronic inflammation. Other helpful herbs and supplements are acetyl-cysteine (NAC), a major support for liver detoxification; silymarin (milk thistle) combined with the supplement berberine; omega-3 fatty acids, which enable cell membranes, including liver cell membranes, to communicate with each other; and vitamin E, which is also vital for gallbladder health and many other functions.

As this chapter makes clear, I also highly recommend individualized weight management vocal analysis as another important step people can take to lose weight. The personal analysis can point you in the appropriate direction to identify your individual weight loss issues and frequencies.

Everyone is biochemically unique. The most extraordinary aspect of Human BioAcoustic Vocal Profiling is the fact that we can individualize every encounter with every client. Unhealthy weight gain can happen for a myriad of reasons. As with any other health issue, the first step is to identify the root causes of the problem. Vocal print analysis can help do this quickly and accurately. From there, a trained Human BioAcoustics practitioner can help support your weight loss needs by providing you with an individualized tone box with a correcting set of frequencies.

Other suggested weight management strategies for fatty liver include:

Dietary Changes: Eliminate refined and artificial sugars, refined carbohydrates, and seed and damaged oils. Genetically modified (GM) or otherwise damaged oils (e.g. canola and other omega-6 seed oils) are a major cause of NAFLD. Also avoid alcohol.

Mediterranean or low-carbohydrate diets are especially effective for helping to reverse NAFLD and stimulating weight loss.

Exercise: Aerobic exercise and resistance (strength) training improve liver fat and insulin sensitivity. For best result, incorporate both aerobics and strength training in your exercise program.

Relieving Spinal Stress: Spinal stress negatively impacts liver function and the function of all other organs in the body. The liver's autonomic innervation (nerve flow stimulation) involves a range of thoracic spinal segments. The primary sympathetic input arises from a segment of the thoracic level of the spine (T7 to T12), and parasympathetic innervation is provided by the vagus nerve. Osteopathic manipulation, chiropractic, and certain types of body work can alleviate spinal stress, as can various stretching exercises.

No matter which weight loss method you choose, many health experts agree that detoxifying a fatty liver is one of the first steps in supporting your body's ability to build and optimally manage fatty acid metabolism.

The Sound Health BioBundles

To manage your weight and body fat, I once again encourage you to embrace the idea of Self-Health by visiting SoundHealthPortal.com. There you will find the BioBundles my team and I have created to monitor your own Human BioAcoustic optimal health factors.

Individual evaluations using weight management BioBundle templates are available to the public at the WorkStation at SoundHealthPortal.com. Join the Guest/Apprentice level and use Weight Management BioBundles to evaluate your weight management issues discussed in this chapter.

To assess your weight issues, skip all the background and go to SoundHealthPortal.com. Record your voice by using the instructions available. Using the appropriate microphone will ensure that your vocal information is accurate. (At SoundHealthOptions.com you will find a list of microphones.)

Once you have saved your voice recording, go to BioBundles and choose WEIGHT MANAGEMENT as an option.

Here is an example of how the next screen on the website will appear.

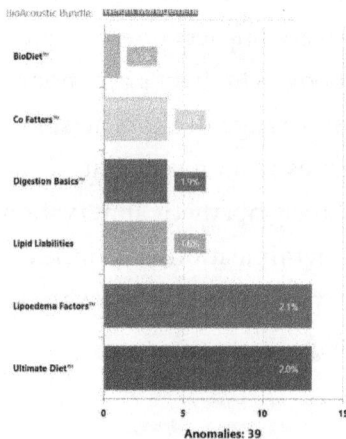
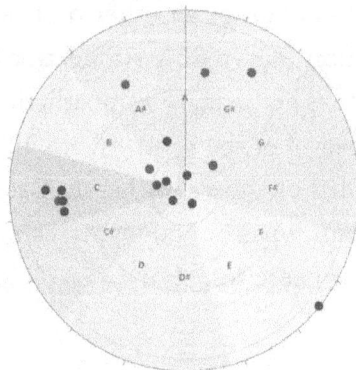

Looking at the left side of the image above, notice which bar has the highest percentage. In this case, it is Lipoedema Factors. which is at 2.1 percent, while Ultimate Diet is at 2 percent.

Lipoedema Factors indicates how the body uses and regulates incoming and stored fat, while Ultimate Diet deals with the biochemistry of metabolism. In both readings, the indications over 2 percent are significant.

The wheel on the right represents corresponding issues. When you are online at the Portal, you can click on any dot within the wheel and it will name the identifying issue. Items in the center of the wheel above are low or missing, and must be addressed. The items on the outer ring, however, are too high, indicating that they are too much of an issue, and also need to be addressed.

From there, when you receive your own analysis, you may want to view a complete report for each of the items that the analysis indicates need your attention.

A preliminary Management Report of Ultimate Diet such as the printout below may show the Frequency Equivalents listing.

Vocal Print

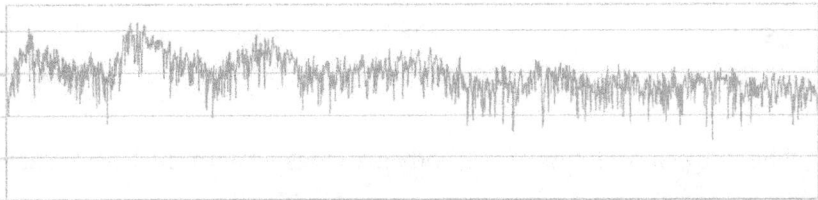

Research Results

				Rank
Alglucerase	Medication	LL	Recombinant glucocerebrosidases - associated with glucose metabolism	1
Cinnamon	Herb	LL	Fat burning spice	1
Glucagon A	Hormone	LL	Helps balance glucose and insulin levels	1
Glucocerebrosidase	Enzyme	LL	aka Imiglucerase (medication)	1

Saturday, November 9, 2024   *results are based on Frequency Equivalents for research purposes only   **Page 1 of 4**

From the desk of: Sharry Practitioner   (740) 698-9119

The numbers on the right indicate the priority of the issue, with those ranked #1 being the most important frequency. "L" indicates an item that is low; LL = Lowest low. Conversely H indicates an item as high, and HH = a Highest High. In both cases (H and HH), that means there is too much of the item.

Once you have these reports, you can work with a Human BioAcoustics practitioner, and also share the reports with your trusted physician and/or other wellness provider.

Conclusion

I love to find answers. And I especially like helping people find their own answers. It is my theory of disease and stress that we are a combination of frequency relationships, with the brain being our central processing unit of control for those frequencies.

If we can identify the stressed mathematical matrix for an individual and provide those sound frequencies to her or him, it will enhance the body's the ability to heal itself. I want everyone to have this opportunity and support. That is why I created the Human BioAcoustic WorkStation for people to create their own vocal print reports.

My issue today is that we don't have enough people trained to do advanced levels of this work. That is why I am providing software and tutorials for the public to learn Human BioAcoustic protocols that will support health.

The frequency matrix of the body provides us with the Rosetta Stone for self-healing. Using a person's own vocal print allows my team and I to customize the individualized sound frequency requirements for optimal form and function related to optimal health.

I hope you will consider learning and using these sound healing techniques to enhance your life, and the lives of your family, friends and others in your community.

CHAPTER 7

VOCAL PROFILING DISTINGUISHES BETWEEN TRUTH AND LIES

"A good man brings good things out of the good
stored up in his heart, and an evil man brings evil
things out of the evil stored up in his heart. For
the mouth speaks what the heart is full of."

~ Luke 6:45

I t is the Truth that humans lie. They lie a lot.

A point to ponder might be, "Why do humans continue to lie?"

"When did lying become a beneficial behavior?"

Animals lie and deceive primarily as a matter of survival. By contrast, often with little or no provocation, humans lie, and many do so on a regular basis. To protect themselves, their reputation, to manipulate and gain advantage, to avoid punishment, for self-preservation, and to appear superior.

On the other hand, if you are a recipient of a lie, the consequences can be devastating, life-altering, and potentially even life-threatening.

Think about the last time someone you cared about lied to you, betrayed you, or attempted to manipulate you using a deliberate falsehood.

You wanted to believe but your lack of faith in your own perceptions put you into a state of conflict. You did not know who or what to believe.

When did we begin to distrust our own perceptions about a person's honesty? Would the world be a better place if deception was impossible? What kind of world would it be if everyone were required to tell the Truth?

What if there was a computer program that could help you discern the Truth? Would you believe such a computer analysis?

There is such a program. It's called the nanoVoice™, and in this chapter, I will explain how the nanoVoice technology I developed can indeed reveal whether anyone is telling the truth or telling a lie. All that is needed to do this is a vocal print of their voice for analysis.

I'll begin by stating this fact: You can lie with your words, but the sounds of your words will give you away 100 percent of the time. People have an intrinsic sense of unease when people are being deceitful because the pitch and jitter of the voice gives away the attempted duplicity. Using the nanoVoice's computerized analysis, anyone who is trained in its use can pick up the nuance of the voice frequencies to ascertain a person's genuine motives.

Have you called an organization only to be told that your voice is being recorded for quality assurance purposes? Chances are you are being screened to determine the emotions behind your motives for calling.

The nanoVoice™

The nanoVoice is computer software that I created in the 1980s when I was a student at the College of Communication at Ohio University. I designed it to help determine if people were truthful. The software evaluates the octaves and frequencies of a person's voice. Years of trial and error have concluded that the voice contains valuable information beyond just the spoken word.

Like a song, each person's voice contains frequencies that can be quantified. The nanoVoice software evaluates six octaves and 12 musical notes gleaned from each person's vocal frequencies. These numeric values should all be connected, and the columns of the print out of the analyses should be balanced, both in color and size.

The energy in your voice creates a matrix which can show your motivation and emotional coherence. This vocal graph below shows a lack of foundation and the person speaking on a naïve, fantasized level. He was likely making up the story he told and leaving out a lot of pertinent information.

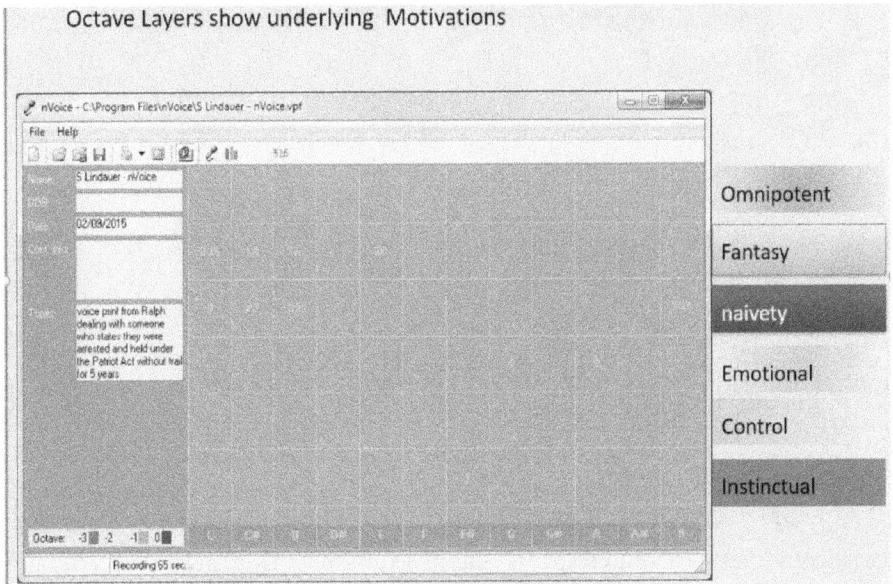

Octave Layers show underlying Motivations

Only you give credibility to the words of others. If you don't think their words contain any truth, you won't be influenced by them.

If you were sitting here in your absolute best red dress and I told, "That is the ugliest yellow dress I have ever seen," you would likely laugh at me, or at least argue that I might be colorblind. But if I said, "Your dress doesn't really look good on you," you may doubt your choice of clothing for the occasion. Only you accepted the truth or untruth about the comment.

Sometimes vocal octaves can be split. The person can actually feel two distinct ways about a topic.

The graph below is a nanoVoice analysis of Jerry Sandusky, who was accused of sexually assaulting a young boy in a locker room when he worked at Penn State. On one level, the analysis showed that he felt such behavior was appropriate (instinctual level) but there was a large gap between his instinctual and fantasy layers, indicating that he had not accepted his own behavior on a personal level. He may have believed that his predatory behavior was normal. It may have happened to him.

He was found guilty.

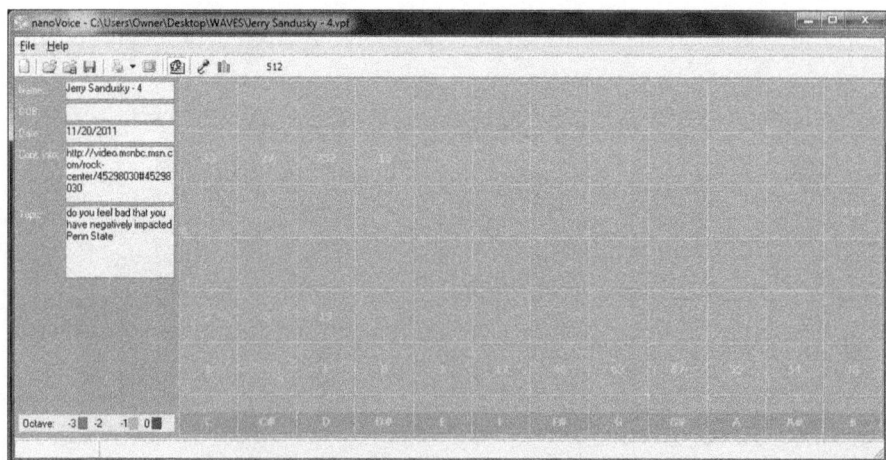

People who are telling the Truth, the whole Truth, have balanced, connected octaves and columns that are shown in their nanoVoice analysis charts. Every box that contains a number is connected to another number-filled box showing the topic coherence of the speaker.

On Feb 24, 2010, then Congressman Ron Paul read a prepared statement to the Senate regarding the US government's assassination of American citizens. Paul reported that on Feb 3, 2010, Dennis Blair, Director of the National Intelligence Committee admitted in open testimony before the Senate that our government has an explicit policy that allows the US government to assassinate American citizens, as well as foreign, at the government's discretion. Below is a nanoVoice evaluation of that speech.

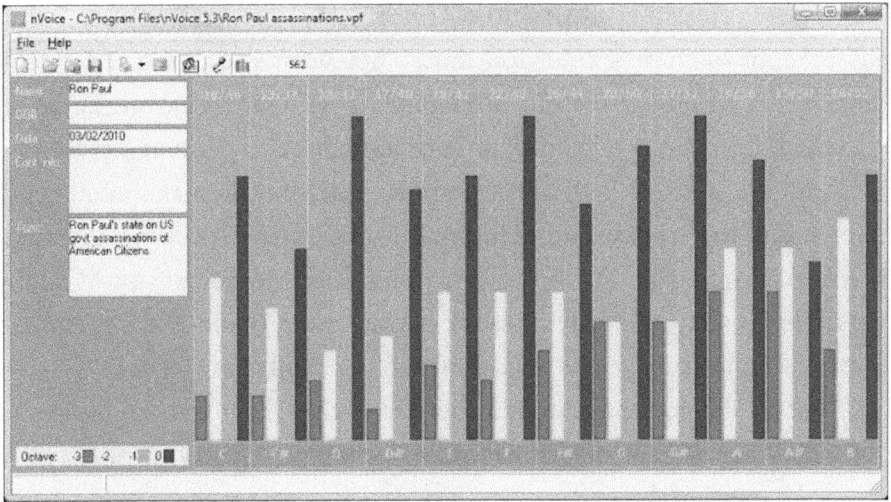

Ron Paul's thoughts are coherent, showing blue (emotions) as his main concern. Green relates to accomplishment, yellow to intellect and red to future concerns.

Analysis of Ron Paul's Vocal Print: Emotions run strong in the need to help others (High Note of "D") which is balanced with the need for that help to be well thought out and useful. A second layer of awareness is planning and doing for long-term outcomes. There is a very balanced mental outlook here. His words are well thought out, balanced, and are spoken for the benefit of all concerned, as shown in the yellow, green and blue balance of the note of "B".

Ron Paul was telling the truth. He has the most truthful vocal print I have ever examined. Since his thwarted run for President in 2008, he has remained a determined patriot and strong supporter of the Constitution, Bill of Rights, and our freedoms.

How to Tell the Truth Tellers From the Liars

Truth tellers want what is best for the most people. The prevaricators (liars) want what is best for themselves and their personal agendas.

Liars share half-truths, withhold information, spin, manipulate, bully, and attempt to control your decisions. They want you to see and accept their truths, like the lover who attempted to betray their partner so he or she could continue having an affair with someone else without disruption.

Honest people tell all of the truth so that you can make intelligent, informed decisions based on all information relevant to the topic that they share, even if it may not be the best thing for them personally. When a person loves you, and really cares about you, they provide all the pertinent information because that is respectful and the right thing to do.

People deserve the truth but sometimes they don't want to hear it.

On the other side of trying to share the truth, you may run into resistance. As an example, one time my husband put on a tie that I didn't think matched the suit he was wearing. I tried to tactfully share my Truth by asking him, "Do you really think that tie matches your suit?" He responded by telling me that I was attempting to tell him how to dress. He denied my perceptions, but he never wore the tie with that suit again. He listened, but he had already made his decision. He was required by his own mind to negate me. His ego was talking.

People who really care about what is best for you will tell you the Truth because they honor your right to make decisions based on reality.

People who lie and distort the truth only care that you see the world their way and, in that situation, will honor their needs, not your own. They want you to serve their purpose.

People who truly care about you don't lie to you to suit their own agenda, nor will they speak against what you know to be appropriate for you.

To me, it is an honor to share my Truth. It doesn't presuppose that you will accept my Truth as your own, however.

What about white lies?

Long ago, I accompanied a friend to an important job interview. When it came time for her to interview, she stood up, did a twirl and asked, "How do I look?" I responded, "Perfect." Had I told her that she had a "run" in her stocking, she likely would have been so self-conscious that she would not have been able to participate in an optimal interview. It was a white lie, done for her benefit. The purpose of the fib was to support her best interests. She got the job.

Sometimes very discreet but hidden information can be ascertained from a vocal graph, based on the reading of each note in the graph.

This is a chart of the overall general meanings of each note.

NOTE CORRELATE CHART

EMOTIONAL		PHYSICAL
Self power, ego, self direct, leader, excitement physically motivated	**C**	Large, thick muscles, heart gross circulation, female reproduction
Champion of justice, fair play, hard on self, stubborn, hard on others as a cover	**C#**	Tendon, ligaments, tissue linings, circulation of digestion, bowel
Self approval, expects reciprocation caretaker, likes to organize, examine and fix self and others	**D**	Liver, gallbladder, pancreas digestion, appetite, production of enzymes and hormones
Information brokers, not apt to share "real" self easily, uses narrative examples to teach	**D#**	Cellular oxygenation, transport of minerals and oxygen to eyes and muscles
Self approval issues, uses words first to convey message and meaning, appreciation	**E**	Wet moist tissues, lungs, eye, nose, bronchial structures diaphragm,
Planner, ability to see flaws in the plan of others, balance between perception and action	**F**	Kidney, environmental allergies prostate, male reproduction, lower back, cranial balance
One who carries out the plans, doer intuitive about the needs of others share and loves wholeheartedly	**F#**	Blood filtering and screening manages mineral balance flow of fluids, nutrients
Game player, likes to mix and manage the physical aspects of life motivated by future events	**G**	Neurotransmitters, balance of minerals and enzymes bone matrix, water balance
Wants to make a difference, likes to help and satisfy others hands on, time conscience	**G#**	Resource maintenance and storage, with C# retrieves nutrients from the bowel
Spiritual, takes care of the needs of others, interprets/acts from within self	**A**	Eye flexibility, electrical issues non-physical issues, resource management, aging
Highly intuitive, reads between the lines, can put aside self for others likes mental games, hurts easily	**A#**	Immune system, adrenal issues with E-allergy related, body detoxification, oxygen regulation
Link between self and universe needs harmony and balance in personal life and occupation	**B**	Subtle circulation, body/mind connection, small body mechanics nerves, body magnetics
Meditative, answers to God's LAW	**B/C**	Body system integration and communication

In the graph below is a nanoVoice analysis of someone telling a story for the future, which is indicated by the red bars. The notes of C#, D, and D# are missing, indicating that information is only being included with some future scenario in mind. This is someone invested in future outcomes but also in what they are withholding.

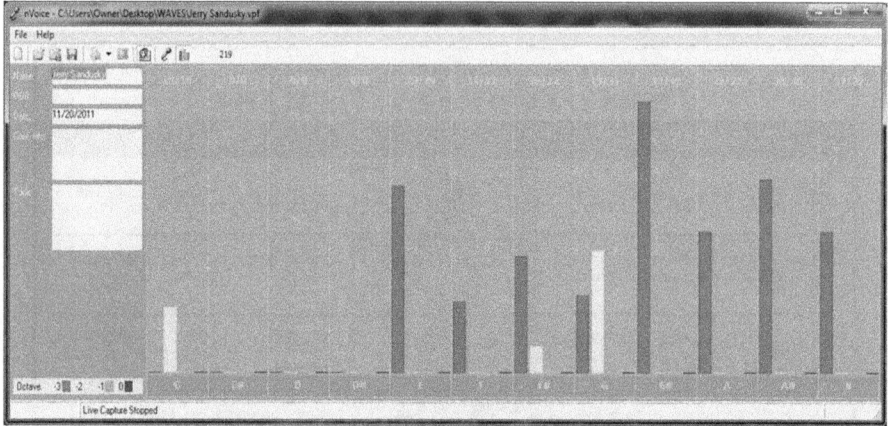

A nanoVoice Analysis of Robert F. Kennedy Jr.

In 2019, I was asked to BioAcoustically evaluate the vocal frequencies of Robert Kennedy Jr. to identify a cause for his stressed speech. Mr. Kennedy appeared to exhibit symptoms of spasmodic dysphonia, a neurological disorder that causes involuntary spasms of the larynx. Human BioAcoustic analysis sees the voice as a holographic representation of the brain. The recurrent laryngeal nerve, connected to the brain, is responsible for voice box function.

Kennedy's vocal print revealed that the frequencies associated with acetylcholinesterase (AChE) were stressed. AChE is an enzyme that catalyzes the breakdown of acetylcholine (ACh) to stop the excitation of a nerve after the transmission of an impulse. AChE is mainly utilized in neuromuscular junctions and synaptic transmission activities. Acetylcholine (ACh) is a compound found throughout the nervous system and functions as a neurotransmitter.

The genetic inefficiency of AChE can cause many issues associated with the use of choline. Inositol, a companion to choline, was also low in Mr. Kennedy's 2019 interviews.

In the 2019 evaluation, the frequencies associated with the posterior cricoarytenoid posterior muscle of his larynx appeared weak. This muscle opens the vocal cords and is also involved in breathing.

I was impressed by the biochemical information gleaned from Kennedy's Human BioAcoustic vocal map but more intrigued by his voice-based nanoVoice Personality Profile. His voice matrix was remarkably similar to that of Dr. Ron Paul, who, as I mentioned above, had the most honest vocal print I had ever reviewed.

I recently used this example of vocal profiling to represent a person who is transparent, honest and awash with integrity. It shows emotions first, then accomplishment, followed by intellect and a solid foundation.

Mr. Kennedy's voice prints from both 2019 and 2023 show similar qualities of accomplishments being primary emotions, secondary intellect, and a strong foundation following. He is a multitasker and a balanced thinker, capable of considering all information needed for a knowledgeable conclusion. Kennedy's voice reveals that he desires leadership transparency but does not believe that it exists in our country today. His words confirm that he believes current leaders attempt to smother the public in narcissistic, self-serving behaviors. He thinks the cover-ups need to be exposed, and that his family must set history straight. He also knows he will likely be threatened.

Kennedy's main concern is intelligent, nonpartisan management of physical priorities. He adroitly uses facts to support his claims. His self-emotions are resilient. I believe he is willing and emotionally capable of bringing freedom and equal justice back to America. His perspective concerning justice is not motivated by personal needs, but by equal justice for everyone. He supports American history as a bastion of freedom equally and wholly distributed to those who deserve protection under the founding principles of democracy.

Kennedy's numeric graph shows equality, knowledge, and transparency. He is unsure if he can win but believes he has the right to try if given the chance to be heard.

The 2023 nanoVoice Evaluation for Kennedy revealed issues with copper support of collagen and elastin. Keep in mind that BioAcoustic Evaluation involves 16 layers of numeric system analysis. The oblique arytenoid, a superficial arytenoid muscle that approximates arytenoid cartilage, shows stress. (The arytenoid muscle is a single muscle of the larynx that passes from one arytenoid cartilage to the opposite arytenoid cartilage. It has oblique and transverse fibers and is affected by the recurrent laryngeal nerve.)

NanoVoice analysis of both Kennedy and Donald Trump revealed that Kennedy has similar ideas about protecting people, America, and our future as does Trump. I predicted that the best ticket could be for the two of them to team up and that happened. Knowing about the personalities and perceptions of people can help predict their behaviors.

Of particular importance, given that he is now in charge of our nation's healthcare, is the nanoVoice report of Kennedy's June 18, 2023 vocal frequencies. What follows is the computerized voice analysis of Kennedy from that time when he was talking about running for President. (**Note:** The analyses provided by the nanoVoice computer are written as if they are directly addressing the person for whom a vocal print has been assessed.)

Points of Importance, Attention, and Consequence: It is hard to understand why people take your peaceful nature as an easy target.

You push yourself and others to finish the job. You love new ideas, which means you can have a project to work on. A sense of belonging is important to you. You may appear to overestimate your value to those around you because your self-approval is solid.

When you think things through from an internal perspective, your philosophical opinions are much appreciated. You challenge the actions of others with good reason. You desire to have information confirmed.

You teach by intellectually adapting your behavior as a good example for others. You appreciate others who recognize your ability to be of service. You have high ideals and expect the same from others.

Sometimes there is a conflict between your ideals and what you want others to think of you. Your highest note is associated with the expression of duty to work and accomplishment. The ability to see the flaws in a plan and make it right resides with this note. Your highest note reflects self-approval and self-worth. Issues of digestion, enzyme, and energy production are associated with this note. Your highest note also associates with the expression of service to humanity and the human spirit. Your feelings and desire to help others reside with this note.

You often have more chores than you can possibly get done. Structure is not required for you to be comfortable. The demands of your life do not leave enough time for you personally. It is essential to consider how your actions influence others. When confronted with what may be untrue, you dare to go to the source and ask for clarification.

You are often haunted by thoughts of what you should have done. You may be caught once in a situation, but not twice, without a proper answer. People who use their position of authority to manipulate others disturb you to the point of action. You often think you should do more than you have time for.

Points of Communication, Complications, and Complaints: Being appreciated for your accomplishments is important to you. You sometimes help others to the detriment of yourself. Your emotions run strong and can influence your health.

You are capable of pushing yourself to get things done. Creating new projects from the ideas you generate is rewarding for you. You take pleasure in changing things for the better.

You have a strong sense of justice, fairness, and truth. Bullies and breaches of trust disturb you at a deep spiritual level.

You can find what you need, so organization is not always necessary. You can get by with what is functional. Your spiritual side may get neglected because of the responsibilities you hold. Taking time for your-self is vital, but you don't always do it. Allowing everything you do to benefit all concerned, even if it stresses you personally, is the best solution for you in the long run.

You wish for the best, which sometimes produces statements of hope instead of facts. You may need more than one opportunity to express your-self to get it right. Meditating about a situation or playing it over in your mind will clarify your stance and help you represent your ideas. Being in stress will likely affect your breathing. You trust until you get hurt, even though making people earn your trust is more logical.

Points of Cooperation, Learning, Opportunity, and Growth: You actively support equal rights in words, deeds, and money when you have it. You can use self-power and self-approval as a potent combination to change opinions. You can be very persuasive when convincing people that their actions and ideas are right or wrong. You have a balanced sense of self-worth.

You can use words to help others find their path. You can go to a deep internal space using self-dialogue. You can talk others into carrying out the details. You can envision a result but do not want to be required to explain everything in detail.

Planning and carrying through your plans are vital aspects of your personality. You plan well and have an intuitive sense of what will work. Others respect your opinions about your projects even though they may argue with your suggestions.

You do for others because they ask, not because they deserve your time. You do for others more quickly than you do for yourself. Helping people grow emotionally and intellectually is rewarding to you.

You have good intentions about bringing your plans to fruition. You sometimes seem disorganized to the casual onlooker.

Your self-approval feeds on appreciation from others. To your detri-ment, you sometimes put the opinions of others ahead of what you think about yourself. You would rather accept criticism than give it. Not knowing the "why" of a situation can cause great concern about your involvement in the outcome.

Your spirituality is often at odds with your physical lot in life. You don't often allow yourself the time to dedicate to your spiritual endeavors. You would like more time to contemplate the universe, humanity, and its place in history. You tend to want to do more than time allows.

Stress can literally take your breath away. You tend to promise more than you have time to deliver. You may not always have the energy to carry out your intentions. You can get excited when talking about an idea but lose interest once you know the outcome.

You are hard-hit at a soul level when justice does not prevail. You actively want to bring spiritual law to your life. Contemplating what you want for your life and those around you will produce peace of spirit. Trusting spirit may come hard for you or too easy because you jump from not questioning to total questioning. A balance between Truth and Spirit must come from within. Listening to others will give you ideas but may not always satisfy you. The best answers come from within.

Vocal Print Analyses of Other Politicians

The use of the nanoVoice can reveal the trustworthiness of anyone so long as an audio of their voice is available. Over the years, I have used it to evaluate various elected leaders. What follow are a few examples of what analyses of their vocal print indicated.

Joe Biden: I analyzed two vocal prints of Joe Biden when he was President, one from 2022 and one from 2024. Both indicate that Biden had within his vocal print the frequencies associated with an anti-dementia agent, most likely Meclofenoxate (also known as Lucidril and centrophenoxine), a nootropic drug. In elderly people, meclofenoxate has been shown to improve performance on certain memory tests. This information could indicate that Biden was on anti-dementia medications while attempting to be the President of the United States. Someone knew this! Who was hiding it from the public, for what purpose, and for how long?

Kamala Harris: When she ran for President, Harris stated that she supported fracking and also that she would ban fracking. Her voice indicated that both positions were true, even though the statements are contradictory. In her case, she was repeating statements that were not part of her own identification, but simply spewing information that she repeated at the behest of someone which wasn't really a part of her own perspective. Kamala's consistent perspective in the majority of her appearances has always been "What can I get out of this?"

In addition, her husband's vocal print revealed that he had absolutely no emotional connection to his statement, "I love her laugh." It was only said to create a justification to get the public to embrace her cackling as something pleasant.

Liz Cheney: The vocal prints of China's President Xi, Joe Biden and Liz Cheney are almost identical, meaning that all three of them have compatible motives for their actions toward the populace. Vocal print analysis showed that the main motive of Liz Chaney for her part in January 6th hearing was revenge against President Trump and not much else.

Hunter Biden: Hunter Biden's vocal prints showed change in his motives, which went from "I was promised that I would be protected" to "I need to be my father's protector."

Barack Obama and Hillary Clinton: Shortly after the Benghazi attack, when the bodies of U.S. personnel were returned home, both Obama's and Hillary Clinton's statements about the cause of those deaths being due to a video were proven to be false. The nanoVoice software concluded that their statements were false two years before their video announcement was revealed publicly as a distortion. Their misinformation was no more than a camouflaged lie.

Donald Trump: Trump's vocal print reveals his current motivations to be a sense that he is carrying out God's mission, feeling that he can do the best job for the people, and his total commitment to Justice as he sees it. But Trump is also withholding a great deal of information that will be released when it will be the most advantageous to him. The information will come out regardless.

My associate, Jocelyn Davies, has compiled a report on the vocal prints of various other American and global leaders and public figures that show their duplicity. It is entitled *The Biggest Liars*, and is available as a free, downloadable PDF document at https://tinyurl.com/bdfkdmdb. It also includes analysis of a few other public figures who are telling the truth.

Honing Your "Spidey Sense" About The Lies You're Being Told

Knowing the motives and perspectives of people can help you be better prepared to make the optimal decisions necessary to live your best life.

Tucker Carlson says that the truth "hums" inside of us like a tuning fork. The only reason we don't act on it is because we have been talked out of it by professional liars. We doubt our own gut instincts! Carlson suggests that we all need to "hone our Spidey senses," and cautions us to remember that misinformation should immediately be labeled as a deliberate lie.

You can lie with words, but the frequencies of your voice will always tell on you. The vocal analysis software of the nanoVoice breaks down the sounds of your voice to reveal hidden personality traits and physical attributes.

We usually know, or at least suspect, when someone is attempting to manipulate us with a lie. We get into trouble when we don't trust our own perceptions or when we allow someone to talk us out of what we believe to be true.

To feel secure, we rely on the truth to help us make decisions that best suit our life goals. Lies cause us to feel betrayed, confused, and manipulated. People who care about what is best for you do not lie to you. People lie to manipulate you, so that you will do what best serves their motivations.

Our world is in chaos now because we have been so thoroughly lied to about our health and other matters over the last few years. Our political system is on the verge of collapse because of the tremendously conflicting lies we have been told by leaders who claim to want to protect us. Those who genuinely care, tell the truth.

From interactions within your family circle, to world politics, Truth must always stand at the forefront of beneficial decisions. Stop depending on your leaders to have your best interests at heart. It is actually up to us, individually, to decide what we accept as supportive, and once we identify the truth from the lies, we can move toward positive action.

If you suspect you have been lied to and want to take action, the following Action Steps for We the People may add to your ability to defend your intrinsic human rights and opinions.

1. Don't allow yourself to be separated or divided from your opinions.
2. Abandon fake media and platforms. De-support those who distort.
3. Evaluate evidence using Truth and Justice as your values.
4. Make sure your vote counts. Insist on election fairness and reform.
5. Support those who cannot be bought, but who might be silenced.
6. Honor Truth and the Rule of Law with full equality for every citizen.
7. Work to improve and enhance our school systems.
8. Evaluate local leaders. Believe their actions, not their words.
9. Know your rights. Read the U.S. Constitution and the Bill of Rights.

10. Challenge rules that are not just and equal for everyone.

11. Insist on Health Autonomy.

12. Remember that Truth and Freedom were the goals of our nation's Founders.

Use the nanoVoice To Find Out What Your Voice Reveals About You

As with all of the other sound healing software and technology that my team and I have developed, my desire for the nanoVoice is to have it included in every household as a tool anyone, with a bit of training, can use to discover more about themselves and the information their voice can reveal. To that end, I offer both a free version of the nanoVoice, as well as a professional version that is very inexpensively priced.

nanoVoice™ is a micro-version of our professional nVoice Personality Profiler™ which uses frequency-based biomarkers within the frequencies of your voice to allow you an enlightening peek into your Secret Self. It can help you understand and solve issues using unconscious levels of awareness. This innovative technology is the forefront of future wellness based on personal biofrequency correlations to emotional, genetic, structural and biochemical information about YOU.

The principles of Human BioAcoustic sound-based therapies originated with the concept that *the brain perceives and generates impulse patterns that can be measured as brain-wave frequencies*. These are delivered to the body by way of nerve pathways. The theory incorporates the assumption that these frequency impulses serve as directives that sustain structural integrity and emotional equilibrium.

When these patterns are disrupted, the *body seeks to reveal the imbalance by manifesting symptoms that can be interpreted as symptoms of disease and stress*. Tapping into these self-healing biological pathways from brain to neuron cell has long been a goal of scientific medical investigations as an approach to provide and promote optimal health.

nanoVoice software is a tool you can use to predict how your body would react based on genomic, environmental and internal stimuli. *Nanovoice was created to spread the word* and show the world what is possible.

nanoVoice is available at the Sound Health Portal, a specialized website designed to facilitate Human BioAcoustic analysis of vocal recordings. It provides detailed, medically related insights based on the vocal patterns, aiding in the assessment and understanding of various health conditions through artificial intelligence and advanced audio analysis techniques.

You can visit https://soundhealthoptions.com/nano-voice to get started using the free version of the nanoVoice Public Voice analysis software.

The nanoVoice software only works on PCs, not Mac (Apple) computers. If you have a Mac (Apple) computer or laptop, you can access this software directly at SoundHealthPortal.com.

For PC users, please see the nanoVoice videos and downloads available at the following website links:

- https://vimeo.com/337832898. Go here to watch the Your Voice Always Tells the Truth video.
- https://vimeo.com/141449982. Go here to download the tutorial on using the nanoVoice software, with the link to download in the description.
- https://vimeo.com/141449984. Go here to watch an additional tutorial on how to use the nanoVoice.
- https://vimeo.com/channels/728774/85155628. Go here to watch six more videos by me explaining the nanoVoice technologies and other aspects of my work.
- https://vimeo.com/112170767. Go here to watch a more in-depth tutorial about the nanoVoice. At this link, you will also find many other educational videos by me related to sound healing.

Instructions For Using the Paid Version of the nanoVoice Software: To begin using the paid version of nanoVoice, you first must have a spreadsheet software like Microsoft Excel for it to work. Then go to https://soundhealthoptions.com/product/nanovoice to purchase and download the nanoVoice software. (**Note:** The professional version is $60.00.)

After you download the nanoVoice software, open it and a Registration box will pop up with a 16 digit code at the top. *Please email that 16 digit code along with the name of the software to SoundHealthInfo@gmail.com in order to receive your serial number needed to run the program. Once you receive the serial number:*

1. Purchase and download nanoVoice™ and the Tiny Nano Manual* (included with your nanoVoice™ software download). Optional: purchase and download Nanovoice Technician BioAcoustic Basics Textbook . (**Please note:** Once you open the Tiny Nano Manual in dropbox.com, please make sure to press "download" under the button located in the top right corner of the page (the button with three dots).

2. Purchase and download Note Correlate Chart and Starter wheel.

3. Watch the instructional video available at https://vimeo.com/142551851.

4. Install the appropriate microphone.

5. Open the program.

6. Select your microphone of your choice and click "OK".

7. Start talking into microphone. (**Note:** The program will automatically stop when it collects 500+ hits.)

8. Save and rename the file you created.

9. Click on the "blue square" to read the report and click "print icon" to print the report.

10. Continue to practice on yourself and others until you are satisfied that you can use the program.

Conclusion

As this chapter makes clear, Human BioAcoustics vocal profiling and assessment using the nanoVoice reveal frequencies of the voice. Subsequent computerized analysis of these frequency notes and octaves are capable of revealing a wealth of information about people, both in terms of their nutritional and overall health status (see the previous chapters in this book), but also other information about them, much of which may be unconscious to them and others. In this regard, the nanoVoice technology can determine whether or not a person is telling the truth or is telling lies.

Imagine how much the state of our nation might change were We the People able to quickly determine if our government leaders, as well as other public figures in positions of authority and responsibility across other segments of our society, were telling us the truth or were lying to us. This is what is possible if enough of use learn how to use the nanoVoice software for both our individual and societal benefit.

The Truth will set us free! And with the nanoVoice, we now have the means to discover it!

CHAPTER 8

HUMAN BIOACOUSTICS AND THE FUTURE OF MEDICINE

Having read this far, you now know how and why Human Bio-Acoustics works and has the potential to revolutionize health care in our nation and around the world.

Although Human BioAcoustic Therapy is certainly not a cure-all, our inventory of unsuccessful outcomes is short. In that vast majority of cases it has proven to be of great benefit. It is most appropriate for none-mergency health conditions, on a predictive, diagnostic, and/or therapeutic basis. I do not recommend it for emergency situations, such as poisoning, traumatic bleeding, broken bones, or situations like heart attack or appendicitis, however. I would never recommend that it be used to set a broken bone, for example, but I would not hesitate to offer it to accelerate healing, reduce pain and swelling, and reduce the recuperation time of such an accident because as an aid to recovery from such circumstances it most definitely helps.

However, even in cases of broken bones, sound therapy may still be helpful. This was demonstrated to me when a woman was brought to my workplace after she fell down some stairs. Her ankle bone was protruding, although not through the skin. My workplace had sound equipment in every room, and I knew from past experience what sounds would set a bone, so I immediately turned on the equipment and had her listen to first-aid bone sound frequencies through our sound presentation speakers. Her pain stopped as her bone reacted immediately to the sound frequencies, and we watched in amazement as the bone moved and set itself. It was an awesome experience, and showcases the great potential for healing that Human BioAcoustics has.

Going Forward

Whenever I am asked about what I foresee as the long-term ramifications of Human BioAcoustics, I first like to address what I foresee in the short-term. The interest in Human BioAcoustics is definitely growing, especially among the health practitioners who are finding out about it. We are even beginning to receive interest by HMO's and so forth.

At the same time, however, many practitioners and organizations are hesitant to explore Human BioAcoustics because it isn't approved by the Food and Drug Administration (FDA) or the American Medical Association, and other, similar organizations. I once had one doctor contact me, for instance, who was very interested in the work I am doing with gout. He asked to see any double-blind studies I had on this. I didn't have any to offer him, because when I contacted the National Institutes of Health (NIH) to inform them of what I was doing, they told me that the best way to facilitate it was through the collection and documentation of case studies, which is what I've done. But when I told the doctor this, he said he couldn't get involved without double-blind studies because it would mean setting himself up to be sued. And, unfortunately, he was right. This is the dilemma that many doctors face when they consider moving beyond their accepted medical training to explore Human BioAcoustics and other healing approaches that have yet to receive widespread, mainstream acceptance despite the fact that numerous documented case histories prove they are valid techniques capable of providing many health benefits.

At the same time, though, I think more and more people are recognizing that organizations like the FDA are hardly infallible. Especially in the aftermath of COVID and the growing number of studies that now document how ineffective the so-called COVID mRNA vaccines were. Not to mention the great harm they have caused so many because of their serious side-effects. This awakening by some physicians and the public at large began well before the pandemic due to previous studies that documented that many of the pharmaceutical drugs the FDA has approved, even when they are properly prescribed and administered, have become one of the leading causes of death in this country.

I think Human BioAcoustics and other positive, non-pharmaceutical technologies will only really become mainstream when the public en masse starts to use their dollars to demand that they become mainstream. This is a trend that is already very much underway.

At the same time, however, I think anybody who is bringing in a new paradigm should expect some resistance. I think it would be a sorry world if everything anybody said was automatically accepted. A certain amount of skepticism is needed to keep us on the path of doing the best we can.

So it's up to me, the person who conceived and developed Human BioAcoustics, to educate people and find a way for them to accept its usefulness. And to do that I have to meet them where they are. Which is exactly why I've set up my educational research center and am training people to bring this out into the world. The more people we train and the more data we collect, the faster we can grow. I also wrote this book for this reason. The more that I can get the word out about the potential Human BioAcoustics and Vocal Profiling have to help people restore their health, the more likely it is that more and more people will want to explore it and, hopefully, also decide to be trained in how to use it for themselves, their family and friends, and others in their community.

I think the promise of Human BioAcoustics in terms of health care will continue to grow. Right now, one of the biggest problems facing us as a nation is the exorbitant costs associated with health care. A significant part of these costs has to do with the inability ability to detect disease early, before it progresses to a more advanced state that is more difficult and more expensive to treat. Human BioAcoustics has much to offer in this area, due to its effectiveness as a predictive and diagnostic tool.

Other areas of high medical costs include rehabilitation expenses, the side-effects of unsuitable medication, and the long-term costs for lingering or incurable disease. These costs can also be ameliorated using Human BioAcoustics. For example, using voice spectral analysis, we have the ability to match medications or nutritional agents to a person's specific needs. We can do this with insulin for diabetes for, for instance. There are many different kinds of insulin, and right now finding the right form to use can be a process of trial and error, sometimes even requiring hospitalization until the proper form is found. We can determine what form to use by looking at which form best matches a person's vocal print.

Just as importantly, Human BioAcoustics can be used to predict states of disease before symptoms manifest. This predictive ability could go a long way towards significantly reducing medical costs by eliminating disease before it occurs. Once people are alerted by the sound frequency technology that they are at risk for a disease condition, they can work with their doctor to proactively shift their bodies into a healthier state. The technology can also guide them on how best to do so, including determining which nutrients they may be deficient in, their stress levels and hormone status, and so forth.

Among the many uses that I foresee for Human BioAcoustics, in terms of it becoming more widely adopted, are:

- Individualized, holistic, predictive, and preventative health screening.
- Drug and nutritional evaluation.
- Nonintrusive blood chemistry screening.
- Nonintrusive temperature control.
- Depiction of disease root causes and disease pathways.
- Identification of viral, bacterial, and fungal infections.
- Identification of stress, paralyzed, or inactive muscles.

All of these benefits are available today, yet, for the most part, are unknown to the majority of doctors and other health care providers, let alone the public.

Among the areas of medicine that I think are most ready for a direct integration of Human BioAcoustics with conventional diagnostic and treatment methods are dietetics, physical therapy and massage, emergency medical technologies, metabolic and genetic disorder screening, and sports medicine. I also think it will prove to be of benefit during space travel, since we can use sound frequencies to exercise muscles during conditions of weightlessness.

Yet another area that I feel Human BioAcoustics could have much value is in addressing bioterrorism attacks from germ and biochemical warfare, which has now become a very serious challenge. Using voice spectral analysis, just as we have been able to identify and reverse infection due to pathogens such as the Epstein Barr virus, Streptococcus and *Chlamydia pneumoniae*, we can also identify the Frequency Equivalents for pathogens such as anthrax and smallpox.

In addition, not only can the Frequency Equivalents of these pathogens be identified, but low frequency analog sound can be used to stimulate the body to eliminate them.

Ultimately, I would like to see Human BioAcoustics used in every facility that deals with people's health in any way—from hospitals, health clinics, and HMO's, to health clubs and health food stores. Should that occur, people everywhere could have the benefit of using it to determine what they need in order to achieve and maintain optimal health, because Human BioAcoustics is a complete system that is very predictive, diagnostic, and therapeutic.

But I also want to stress that health care is only one area for which Human BioAcoustics holds great value. Now that the foundation work has been completed, I'm realizing that the possibilities for it are far more extensive than I previously imagined. Among the other areas for which preliminary research indicates that Human BioAcoustics is feasible are medical monitoring through voice spectral analysis over the telephone, the individuation of medications to reduce side-effect risk, drug and chemical screening for law enforcement agencies, large area pest control without environmental side-effects, nontoxic fertilization, food preservation, and reversal of environmental pollution.

Other uses, some of which I've already shared with you in previous chapters, include:

- Support for predictive, and reversals of sports injuries and trauma.
- Elimination of fibromyalgia pain.
- Elimination of muscle pain from overwork or exercise.
- Reversals of diseases previously thought incurable, such as multiple sclerosis (MS).
- Noninvasive, inexpensive, fast and efficient biochemical evaluation.
- Monitoring of pregnancy and as a predictor of actual labor readiness.
- Predictive biological system analysis for insurance and medical modeling.

Finding root cause of issues such as mitochondrial disorders, allergies, diabetes, immune deficiencies, arthritis, heart disease, macular degeneration, hormonal disorders, and genetic syndromes.

Individualizations of medications and medical modeling to reduce side-effects.

Medical monitoring through voice spectral analysis via telephone, computer, and satellite for mobile medicine in space or on the battlefield.

Mobile medicine diagnostics and treatment drug and chemical screening for law enforcement agencies.

Diagnosis of large structures through vocal profiling of inhabitants.

Evaluation of transmit systems via vocal profiling of users.

Large area pest control as an insect and rodent repellent without creating environmental side-effects. Potentially, it could even be used to repel sharks near beaches.

As a non-toxic fertilizer.

Food preservation through low frequency presentation.

Detection and reversal of environmental pollutants.

Detection of environmental pathogens as future medicine by the development of predictive templates of disease and genetic traits.

The development of designated sound presentation devices that could be used individually to eliminate various conditions, such as the Dedicated Tone Boxes that are already available to help manage back pain, muscle cramps, and gout, and more (see Chapter 5).

And then there is the potential Human BioAcoustic has via its patented nanoVoice Vocal Profiling analysis to enable law enforcement agencies, the judicial system, corporations, and the public at large to quickly determine whether or not what is being presented to them by others is the truth or lies. Just imagine the changes that would occur for the better were the nanoVoice widely available to analyze vocal prints of our politicians and other leaders. Lying, by necessity, would have to be jettisoned by them if they wished to remain in power, if their words could be screened for the truth

As I often say about Human BioAcoustics, the sky's the limit in terms of all that it might achieve in the future.

Become A Human BioAcoustic Practitioner

It's long been a dream of mind that there be as least one practitioner of Human BioAcoustics in every community across the United States and in communities in other countries, as well. Ideally, I would love to see Sound Health practitioners in every home, and a Human BioAcoustics Center in each community. What a difference that would make in the health of families, communities, and our nation!

To this end, I have done all that I can to make the Sound Health technologies my team and I have developed readily available to everyone. In some cases, they are offered for free, such as the use of the nanoVoice that you learned about in Chapter 7, which anyone can use to obtain a computerized analysis of their vocal print simply by making a recording of their voice online at www.soundhealthportal.com.

I have also done all that I can to make training available to anyone who is interested in learning how to learn how to offer various Human BioAcoustic services, starting with a free 15-day trial for the first tier of the training.

There are three levels to the training, each of which is available to anyone who is interested in becoming a Human BioAcoustic practitioner, with the third level ending in a certification process that designates those who complete this level to be certified practitioners capable of offering the widest range of services using my proprietary technologies.

The three levels are training are Guest/Apprentice, Technician, and Practitioner.

Guest/Apprentice (Level One): The Guest/Apprentice Level is designed to inform you about Sound Health's leading-edge research and why you and how you can be involved with. This course will also introduce you to our online WorkStation, otherwise known as The Portal (www.soundhealth-portal.com). It is available for free for the first 15 days, and afterward you can continue to access it for a monthly subscription fee of $19.95 each month. A subscription includes unlimited use of the nanoVoice II™, Nutrition Provider™, Muscle Management™ and much more. This level of training is self-directed and includes access to my Institute's proprietary software.

As an Apprentice, you will be able to use the Sound Health Portal, discover the power of Human BioAcoustics and Sound Health, and develop the skills that are a prerequisite to be a Sound Health Technician. You will also have access to additional Sound Health Templates, Network within the Sound Health Family, and receive alerts for offers and promotions from the Institute.

Technician (Level Two): This level of training incorporates the basics of Human BioAcoustic Vocal Profiling. Within it, you will learn how to take a vocal print, identify imbalances in the voice using propriety software, generate reports, evaluate relevance, and work with wave file architectures to create client reports.

This training is a prerequisite for the Practitioner Training (Level Three) offered to health care professionals and for those who want to prepare to become a Human BioAcoustic Practitioner. It is designed to acquaint students with the introduction and background of Human BioAcoustic Biology. Using individualized self-instruction and step-by-step guidelines, the information in this course will prepare students to perform computerized vocal assessments and create management reports. It is also designed to further acquaint students with the Sound Health online work station (Portal).

During the course of this training, participants have the opportunity to learn: to generate reports using the Sound Health Portal, to evaluate relevance, and to work with wave file architectures. Once fully trained, a Human BioAcoustic Technician can generate a report in about 15–20 minutes. Fully trained Human BioAcoustic Technicians typically charge $30–$50 per report and can purchase Sound Health products at wholesale prices and Public Version software.

This training is also offered online and can be taken at any time, with students learning at the pace that is best for each of them.

Included in this training:

- Software Registration (1 Year)
- All of the BioBundles created by the Institute.
- Software Included Abacus, Muscles & Nutrition Consultant
- Tools and Solutions for Self Help
- Information on how to start a business or become a trainer.
- The cost of the Technician training course is $450.00.

Practitioner (Level Three): The Practitioner Training level is offered via group sessions for organizations, and as a one-on-one course with me for busy professionals. Each course is individualized for the specific needs of each participant and includes six to eight two-hour sessions. The training is a combination of self-paced and personal sessions, all of which are conducted online with me. Participants move through specific Portal protocols to prepare themselves to deal with the professional aspects and responsibilities of being a Human BioAcoustic Provider. Access to all of the math-based sound frequencies are included, as are frequency-based BioMarkers. Participants learn to use basic Human BioAcoustic equipment. This training level is for people who want to do research and training. Participants may be eligible for additional Portal participation.

Participants in this training have access to dozens of high level Sound Health Templates and other professional level materials, are provided with a Starter Kit that includes all Technician Start Kit Templates, and on taught how to use the most precise sensitivity setting during frequency analysis, with the highest level data processing.

At present, the Practitioner Training is available at a cost of $4400.00, and includes all necessary equipment and Portal access and storage for an additional $34.95 per month.

Practitioner Certification: Each person who takes the Practitioner Training has to present my team and me with a series of case studies, which we then evaluate. Only when we are satisfied with their competency do we certify them, and they then must renew their certification each year, since the research into Human BioAcoustics is still unfolding.

People interested in experiencing Human BioAcoustics need to know they should only work with certified practitioners, whom they can locate by contacting our office or by visiting our website. That way they can be assured of working with someone who knows what he is doing.

Benefits of Participating in Human BioAcoustic Courses

- Save time by mathematically accessing root causes
- Noninvasive mobile assessments
- Mathematically support optimal predictive form and function
- Explore the protocols of Math and Medicine
- Portal storage cache for client records and comparison
- Classes offered online in individual sessions and groups
- BioMarker/BioBundle root cause protocols on the Portal

- System Management
- 300+ templates via 200,000 BioMarker entries
- 24/7 Online WorkStation (the Portal)
- Portal reference and tutorials included
- Metabolic mapping
- Study with me, the Pioneer of Human BioAcoustics.

Conclusion

One of the primary messages I want people to know about my work is that the state of your health may be found in the sound of your voice. The protocols of Human BioAcoustics offer an accurate and noninvasive use of frequencies and architectures found in the human voice spectrum to readily identify the innate mathematical BioMarkers that have been shown to be a holographic representation of a person's physical and emotional health status. As such, Human BioAcoustic Biology has the potential to save people time and resources when it comes to their health.

The research that is continually being conducted by the Institute of BioAcoustic Biology and Sound Health is at the forefront of a new approach to medicine, one that is creating a doorway to the next dimension of the health revolution. The Sound Health techniques of using math as a basis of wellbeing may be the means of restoring our intrinsic right to Self-Health.

Remember this:
Whoever controls health controls the quality of life.
If we can BioAcoustically continue to manage our health, we have dominion over it. The Institute is the recognized leader of the cutting edge of Vocal Profiling BioMarkers, and we intend to remain in that position as we continue to research and develop innovative products and protocols to enhance life through sound-frequency applications. This will allow Human BioAcoustics Self-Health care to become more distinguished, affordable, effective, and available by increasing our network of education

and training in partnership with innovative schools and organizations. I encourage everyone reading this book to join me in this mission by taking advantage of the Institute's trainings and product offerings so that you can empower yourself, your family, friends, and fellow members of your community to achieve and maintain more optimal levels of health and well-being.

CONCLUSION

At its core, bioacoustics is the science of how sound affects living organisms. But as you've now learned after reading this far, Human BioAcoustics is far more profound than that. It is a groundbreaking approach to decoding a person's voice to analyze the body's internal state. Your voice isn't just a tool for communication. It's literally a diagnostic instrument when properly analyzed using the Human BioAcoustic technology my team and I have developed. It's a map, and a frequency fingerprint of the body in real-time.

As the information in this book makes clear, your voice is a holographic representation of your body; it reflects everything. Every cell in the human body vibrates at a specific frequency. Organs, tissues, bones, even our emotions have unique vibrational signatures. When the body is in balance, these frequencies harmonize. When disease or dysfunction occurs, those frequencies become distorted—either too high, too low, or missing altogether.

Long ago, I realized that these changes weren't abstract. They could not only be heard, they could be measured. Recognizing this, I began applying Fast Fourier Transform (FFT) technology to voice recordings, breaking them down into spectral components that created a visual graph of the frequencies present in a person's voice.

Peaks and valleys in this voiceprint revealed surprising insights: a magnesium deficiency here, a liver overload there, emotional trauma nested in the resonance of the throat. Each voiceprint is like a musical score of the body's symphony. Or its disharmony. By reading this "score", practitioners could predict imbalances before symptoms ever became visible, allowing for preemptive, personalized wellness strategies. Health isn't guesswork. The voice gives us the answers if we're willing to listen.

But diagnosis is only one part of the equation. Once a problem frequency is identified, a corresponding corrective tone can be calculated and delivered back to the body using a tone generator. These tones aren't random notes. They are mathematically calibrated to rebalance the body's vibrational structure. The sound frequency protocols I've developed are based on this concept.

One of the most attractive elements of Human BioAcoustics is how easy it is to use and gain benefit from. Once a person's vocal print has been analyzed by the proprietary computerized programs available through the Institute that I founded, all that is necessary is for a person to sit in a quiet space, listening through headphones to the precise sound frequencies their bodies required to create optimal form and function. Some sessions last only 15 minutes; others take longer. Though the effects may often be subtle at first, they invariably produce a sense of calm, and improved focus. Then, with consistent daily listening for the individual prescribed time for each session, more apparent, measurable changes occur. Typically, pain subsides, energy increases, and a person's emotional regulation improves.

Human BioAcoustics bridges multiple disciplines, combining principles from physics, neurology, biochemistry, music theory, and systems biology. And unlike many other forms of healthcare, it was noninvasive, drug-free, and completely individualized. Your voice is your medicine cabinet. Human BioAcoustics just gives you the key to open it.

In the course of my work and research, I also discovered that emotional states can be detected in the voice. Anxiety, depression, grief, and joy all leave distinct imprints. This fact has enormous implications, not just for health, but for education, relationships, and even criminal justice. Could lie detection be replaced by vibrational honesty via the nanoVoice technology you learned about in Chapter 7? Can schoolchildren be given emotional support based on subtle changes in their voice? I believe the answers to such questions is a resounding Yes, and my research bears this out. The possibilities for Human BioAcoustics stretch far beyond medicine.

What began as an intuitive gift that I was born with has become a repeatable process. A system and field rooted in ancient understandings of sound and refined through the lens of modern technology. Human BioAcoustics asks us to reconsider everything we think we know about health. It invites us to listen not just to symptoms, but to the signals beneath them. It empowers us to tune in to ourselves, our needs, and our potential for healing through resonance.

The idea is radical, yet disarmingly simple: Every organ, every cell, every biological system operates at a specific resonant frequency. When these frequencies are disrupted—by stress, toxins, trauma, or deficiency—imbalance arises. By identifying those imbalances by analyzing the voice, we can restore harmony by delivering corrective sound frequencies in place of chemicals or surgery. Frequencies are the medicine of the future—accessible, precise, and profoundly personal.

Using data gathered from thousands of vocal recordings, I have mapped frequency correlations to numerous specific biological functions. I discovered that certain frequency ranges aligned with nutrients like magnesium, others with hormones like estrogen, and still others with neurotransmitters like serotonin. I wasn't just hearing pitch. I was decoding the vibrational blueprints of the body.

With this knowledge, I developed custom tone generators and frequency delivery systems that provide precision-calculated, frequency-specific interventions. The frequencies may sound like simple tones, but these tones were carefully chosen to resonate with what a person's body needed most. I call this method Sound Health—the use of targeted sound frequencies to restore the body's natural vibrational order.

By identifying emotional signatures in the voice, I created protocols not only for physical healing but for emotional release. As my work progressed, I, along with other Human BioAcoustic practitioners I trained, began using frequency protocols for weight loss, learning disorders, immune support, and even addiction recovery. The results varied, but patterns emerged.

Certain tones helped regulate appetite. Others boosted focus in children with ADHD. The voice became both a diagnostic map and a healing compass. Frequencies were no longer abstract vibrations. They were actionable data that offered a way to speak directly to the body in its own language. And in doing so, they reminded people of something powerful: Healing doesn't always come from the outside. Sometimes, it comes from listening inward and playing the right note.

Let me add here that Human BioAcoustics was never meant to replace medicine. But, rather, to evolve it, because sound doesn't threaten medicine. It completes it.

And so, what began for me as a lonely journey into sound has become a quiet revolution, one that was beginning to echo beyond the walls of my lab, challenging the boundaries of what health could be and how we choose to hear it.

My team and I have documented thousands of cases of significant health improvements achieved by Human BioAcoustic sessions. We've built a growing library of case studies that support what the data had already begun to prove years ago: Vocal profiling can detect issues before symptoms appear, and frequency-based interventions can shift outcomes.

Over the years, various communities started adopting the tools. Parents ran voiceprints on their children at home. Teachers used tonal balancing to improve focus and behavior in classrooms. Therapists integrated sound frequency sessions into trauma recovery programs. Farmers even began experimenting with the method on livestock, reporting calmer, healthier animals. Online, an entire ecosystem bloomed into forums where users shared experiences, asked questions, and helped fine-tune protocols for everything from chronic fatigue to emotional burnout. What once lived in the margins of alternative medicine was now growing roots in everyday life. People are waking up to the fact that healing doesn't have to hurt. It can hum. And thanks to Human BioAcoustics, it is now doing just that. One tone, one person, one success story at a time.

But I know that health revolution I am doing my part to help bring about is only as strong as the people who carry it forward. From the beginning, my mission wasn't just to heal—it was to teach others how to listen, how to analyze, and how to apply the principles of Human BioAcoustics in the real world. I recognize that when you teach someone to hear their body, you give them back their power. Human BioAcoustics isn't just a system. It's a language. And we're teaching the world to speak it.

I also made a conscious decision to avoid the exclusivity seen in many medical and alternative training programs. I want my knowledge to remain open-source. To this end, I launched an online library of research papers, instructional videos, frequency databases, and free software tools in order to make my life's work accessible to anyone with curiosity and a computer. At my Institute, students can take part in live voiceprint assessments, participate in client sessions, and co-develop new techniques. It's become a learning lab, a mentorship space, and a community incubator all in one. Many students described their experience not just as educational, but transformational.

I've also initiated programs to bring Human BioAcoustics into K–12 education. I believe that if children could be taught to understand their own emotional and physical signals early in life, they'd grow up more balanced, self-aware, and resilient. Pilot projects in this regard have shown great promise. Students used simple apps to check their own vocal patterns. Teachers used frequency tones to calm hyperactivity or support focus before exams.

Even in the face of technological skepticism, I remain a fierce advocate for democratizing access to sound-based health. I'm not trying to create a guru-driven empire. I'm trying to build a global chorus of informed voices. My work is not about creating followers. It's about awakening leaders—people who can hear the truth in a whisper and turn it into wellness.

As I continue to maintain, "The future of medicine is frequency. And the future is now." With the rise of artificial intelligence, biofeedback systems, and wearable health tech, I envision a world where everyone can have access to personalized, frequency-based diagnostics right from their phone or smart device.

Imagine waking up, speaking into an app, and receiving a comprehensive report about your body's current nutritional, hormonal, and emotional status just from your voice. That's not a fantasy. It's already happening. The software that began as rough, analog recordings and hand-drawn waveforms is now being refined into AI-powered tools capable of generating real-time vocal analysis. These tools don't just identify problems. They suggest personalized sound protocols that users can stream immediately, empowering people to take charge of their wellness on a daily basis.

At my Institute, the next generation of researchers, practitioners, and developers continue to build on my work. They're exploring applications for sports optimization, dementia support, addiction recovery, prenatal care, and even interspecies communication. Some are studying how tones can influence gene expression, opening doors to epigenetic applications of sound therapy.

Our voice is the most underutilized health monitor we possess. It is a biometric signature, a signal flare from our cells, a language of wellness that transcends lab reports. Every pitch, every wobble, every whisper carries biological truth. Health is not outside of us. It's within us, waiting to be heard. And when you understand the language of the body, you no longer guess. You know.

As more people experience the profound shifts that come from sound frequency-based wellness, my hope is that the Human BioAcoustic movement will continue to grow, leading to a global awakening. But beyond the science, beyond the technology, there remains the heartbeat of what I desire most for everyone: empowerment. When people learn to listen to their own voice—not metaphorically, but literally—they reconnect with an ancient intelligence. They remember that they are not broken. They are simply out of tune.

This is more than a story. It's a sound wave rippling through history. And now, you are part of it. The revolution will not be televised. It will be audible. In every restored voice, every harmonic balance, every healed life. Your voice is your medicine. Your resonance is your revolution. Learn to use it and soar!

RESOURCES

Institute of BioAcoustic Biology and Sound Health
5151 Alton Street
Albany, OH 45710
(740) 698-9119

For more information about Human BioAcoustics and the work of Sharry Edwards, including classes and training, nanoVoice, clinical services, blog articles, to sign up to join Sharry's email list, and more, please visit the following websites:

www.soundhealthoptions.com

This is the Institute of BioAcoustic Biology and Sound Health's main website for the public. Learn more about the company and Sharry Edwards, register for the Institute's 2-Day and 5-Day classes, find out more about their upcoming events and news, and locate a Human BioAcoustic Practitioner near you

www.soundhealthportal.com

This is Institute's Online WorkStation, otherwise known as "The Portal." Here you can create an account where you can use the Institute's proprietary software online and store your data. The Institute offers a 15 day free trial for those who are interested in a test run.

www.bioacousticsolutions.net

This website also provides information about the Institute and Sharry Edward's ongoing research. It is primarily intended for professional practitioners.

REFERENCES

Acoustic Brainwave Entrainment with Binaural Beats. "Resonant entrainment of oscillating systems". Retrieved January, 2004, from http://neuroacoustic.org/articles/articlebinaural.htm 32 Copyright, 2013 by Sharry Edwards – All Rights Reserved www.SoundHealthOptions. com.

Anomalous Vocal Patterns used to Detect Biometric Expressions Relating to Structural Integrity and States of Health. Sharry Edwards, MEd. Sound Health Research Institute [a registered 501(c)(3)] (www. soundhealthresearch.org). Albany, OH.

Atkinson, M., McCraty, R., & Tomasino, D. (Comps.). *Science of the Heart: Research Overview and Summaries.* Retrieved 2002, from http://heartmath.org/research

Publication No. 01-001. HeartMath Institute. Boulder Creek, CA.

Bailey, A. (1953). *The Basic Causes of Disease. In Esoteric Healing.* NY, NY: Lucis Trust.

Berard, MD, G., & Monnier-Clay, S. (1993). *Hearing Equals Behavior* (B. Rimland, Trans.). New Canaan, CT: Keats Publishing.

BioAcoustics In Action [Brochure]. (1999). Albany, Ohio: Sound Health.

Butterworth, B. (1999). *What Counts: How Every Brain is Hardwired for Math.* Pasadena, CA: Free Press.

Boaz, N. T. (1977). *Eco Homo: How the Human Being Emerged for the Cataclysmic History of the Earth.* NY, NY: Basic Books.

Campbell, D. (1999). High Performance. *ADVANCE for Speech-Language Pathologists and Audiologists*, May 31.

Charous, S. J., Kempster, G., Manders, E., & Ristanovic, R. (2001). The effect of vagal nerve stimulation on voice. *Laryngoscope*, Nov, 2028-31.

Cowan, J. (1994). *Handbook of Environmental Acoustics*. NY, NY: Van Nostrand Reinhold.

Davis, D. (2002). BioAcoustic Voiceprint Frequencies & Otoacoustic Emissions. Davis Center. Presented at the American Academy of Audiology Convention. April 19, 2002.

Devlin, K. J. (2001). *The Math Gene*. NY, NY: Basic Books.

Duke Encyclopedia of New Medicine, 2006, compiled by the Center for Integrative Medicine at Duke University, pp 566.

Eco, Umberto. (2002). *Art and Beauty in the Middle Ages*. New Haven, Connecticut: Yale University Press.

Edwards, S. (2006). *Exploring sound-based biology: An introduction to human bioacoustics*. BioAcoustic Research Institute.

Edwards, S. (2010). Vocal profiling and frequency-based diagnostics. *Journal of Complementary and Integrative Medicine.* 7(2):101–110.

Faksova K, Walsh D, Jiang Y, Griffin J, et al. COVID-19 vaccines and adverse events of special interest: A multinational Global Vaccine Data Network (GVDN) cohort study of 99 million vaccinated individuals. *Vaccine*. 2024 Apr 2;42(9):2200-2211.

Franke, Sylvia. *The Tree of Life and the Holy Grail.* (2007). East Sussex, UK: Temple Lodge Publishing, Ltd.

Galileo, G. (1623). *Book of Nature.* Bellosguardo, Italy: Concepts translated by Joseph C. Pitt (*Galileo, Human Knowledge, and the Book of Nature* (1992) Kluwer Academic publishers.

Gray, H. & Clemente, C. D. (1986) *Gray's Anatomy of the Human Body.* Lea & Febiger.

Herivel, J. (1975). *Joseph Fourier: The Man and the Physicist.* Oxford.

Holl, R. (1996). Health Problems Displayed in Voice Patterns. *Alternative Health Practitioner,* 2 No 3, Fall/Winter.

Horowitz, L. G. (1999). *Healing Codes For The Biological Apocalypse.* Tetrahedron Publishing Group.

Hunt, V. (1996). *Infinite Mind: Science of Human Vibrations of Consciousness.* Mailbu, California: Mailbu Publishing.

James, E. (2015). The voiceprint of health: A review of bioacoustic technologies. *Alternative Therapies in Health and Medicine.* 21(5): 34–41.

Kersing, W., Dejonckere, P. H., Buschman, H. P., & van der As, H. E. (2002). Laryngeal and vocal changes during vagus nerve stimulation in epileptic patients. *Voice,* June, 251-7.

Landau E. Symphony of stars: The science of stellar sound waves. Jul 30, 2018. https://science.nasa.gov/universe/exoplanets/symphony-of-stars-the-science-of-stellar-sound-waves

Lipton, B. H. (2005). *The Biology Of Belief: Unleashing The Power Of Consciousness, Matter & Miracles.* Hay House.

Ohno, M. (1986). The all pervasive principle of repetitious recurrence governs not only coding sequence construction but also human endeavor in musical composition. *Immunogenetics,* 24[2], 71-78.

Orlikoff, R. F. (1988). The relationship of age and cardiovascular health to certain acoustic characteristics of male voices. *Speech Hear Res,* June 31[2], 207-11. PMID: 2232763.

Oschman, J. L. (2000). *Energy Medicine: The Scientific Truth.* NY, NY: Churchill Livingstone.

Pert, Candace. (1997). *Molecules of Emotion.* New York, New York: Scribner.

Rake, M. (2000). A Voice for All Ages. Perspectives, Autumn/Winter. *Alumni Magazine for Ohio University,* Athens, Ohio 45701.

Ramig, L. A., & Ringel, R. L. (1983). Effects of physiological aging on selected acoustic characteristics of voice. *Speech Hear Res,* March 26[1], 22-30.

Santos, P. M. (2003). Evaluation of laryngeal function after implantation of the vagus nerve stimulation device. *Orolaryngol Head Neck Surgery,* 129[3], 269-73.

Schultz, I. (1976). Importance of the nonverbal characteristics of the speech signal for evaluating the mental and physical state of a pilot [1976PMID:1011788]. *Pub Med.*

Schwarts, MD, D., Howe, C., & Purves, D. (2003). The Statistical Structure of Human Speech Sounds Predicts Musical Universals. *Journal of Neuroscience*, 23[18], 7160-7168.

Science Proves Feeling Good Grows on You. Retrieved 2004, from http://www.universal-tao.com/article/science.html.

Stripe, B & Rezaei, M. (1998). Single Molecule Vibrational Spectroscopy and Microscopy. *Science*, June.

Tiller, W. A. (1997). *Science and Human Transformation: Subtle Energies, Intentionality and Consciousness.* Walnut Creek, CA: Pavior Publishing.

Tomatis, A. (1991). The Conscious Ear: My Life Of Transformation Through Listening. Station Hill Press.

Weiss, Piero and Taruskin, Richard. *Music in the Western World*, 2nd edition. Cengage Learning, Independence, KY. 2007.

Wilson-Pauwels, E., Akesson, & P., Stewart. (1988). *Cranial Nerves: Anatomy and Clinical Comments.* Toronto/Philadelphia: B.C. Decker Inc.

Wolfe, D. (2018). *Frequency Healing: A New Frontier In Health And Medicine.* Longevity Press.

University of Chicago Hospital. Retrieved 2003, from www.uchospitals.edu/areas/epilepsy/vagus.html

Xue, S., & Deliyski, D. (2001). Effects of Aging on Selected Acoustic Voice Parameters of Elderly Speakers: Preliminary Normative Data. *Educational Gerontology*, 21, 159-168.

ACKNOWLEDGMENTS

I have known Larry Trivieri Jr for over twenty years, ever since he included my research in two of his first books – *Alternative Medicine: the Definitive Guide* and *Health on the Edge*. He was our first national acknowledgement. His continued support gave me the courage to move forward even though the uphill climb was very draining. Without him, this book would not have been possible both emotionally and physically. Thank you Larry for your continued support and faith in this cosmic adventure.

To Mortonette who was always there with ideas and friendship even though we were often continents apart.

To my family members, both near and far, who endured many hours of experimentation and abandonment without complaint or judgment

To the hundreds of pioneers who volunteered their vocal profiles and information that allowed this work to grow. Special thanks to Sally, Bonnie, Debra and Becky for your unwavering support and commitment to this work early on.

ABOUT SHARRY EDWARDS—
AN APPRECIATION BY LARRY
TRIVIERI JR

"Healing isn't magic; it's mathematics.
It's physics. It's frequency."

~ Sharry Edwards

In my long career as an investigator of, and writer about, cutting edge healing methods, I've had the great fortune to meet literally hundreds of truly exceptional healers and visionaries. I consider Sharry Edwards, MEd, to be among the very best of them. The work that she is doing in the field of sound therapy is to me one of the most important breakthroughs in the entire field of healing, both conventional and holistic.

Sharry is the recognized leader in the emerging field of Human BioAcoustic Vocal Profiling. She pioneered and developed the theories that have been recognized and incorporated by many health care researchers as they attempt to improve our present health care system using frequency based modalities. Throughout her long and illustrative career, Sharry has always strived to establish Self Health as a basic human right. She is the Architect of the Mathematical Matrix for Sound Health, and received the New Scientist of the Year Award from The International Association of New Science (IANS) in 2001. She is also a recipient of the prestigious 2002 O. Spurgeon English Humanitarian Award from Temple University.

Sharry's pioneering achievements are all the more remarkable when you consider her background. She was born and raised by her adoptive parents in rural Ohio, a region at the time in which many lived in poverty. During her childhood, Sharry's home lacked electricity, central heating, running water, and even an indoor toilet. Despite these obstacles and the fact that her early formal education was severely limited, Sharry became the first person in her family to finish high school, and then went on to achieve a college degree.

In Sharry's words, "I was raised in Southeastern Ohio when education was not a priority. It took me twelve years to finish my undergraduate degree a few courses at a time. I was a working mother of three small children but I did it. I went on to finish a Master's and was admitted to a doctoral program at Ohio University, but no formal education could have prepared me for developing the field of Human BioAcoustics."

From the time she was a child, Sharry grew up hearing what others could not. Voices, yes—but also frequencies. Her perception extended into a realm most people never sense: The subtle variances in pitch, tone, and vibration that carry biological meaning. Where others simply listened to sound, Sharry experienced it as a language—one that spoke of health, emotion, and internal imbalances.

"I never just heard voices. I heard information, imbalance, potential," she says.

When still a child, Sharry often startled others by pointing out oddities in their voices or predicting illnesses before symptoms became visible. Her family, though bewildered at times, began to notice that her insights were more than coincidence. She would say, "Grandma's voice sounds tired today," and a few days later, Grandma would be in bed with the flu.

While these observations were dismissed by many as childish or imaginative, they were seeds of something much deeper. Growing up in a region rich in oral tradition and folk remedies, Sharry's abilities were sometimes seen as a mystical gift—though not always with warmth. Neighbors whispered. Teachers raised eyebrows. Some were fascinated; others were unnerved.

But Sharry remained undeterred. Even at a young age, she understood that what she heard wasn't magic—it was math. It was structure. It was signal.

During her teenage years, Sharry had developed a deep love for the sounds of nature and people at play and work, but also frustration that no one seemed to grasp what she was hearing. She kept notebooks full of observations about voice fluctuations and people's health, often drawing rudimentary sound waves by hand. She became obsessed with the question: What if this isn't imagination? What if there's something measurable happening here?

To find answers, she began performing small experiments. With an old cassette recorder and a tuning fork, she documented the voices of friends and family members over time. She noticed that when someone was stressed, the upper frequencies in their voice would become jagged or disappear entirely. When someone was joyful, their vocal pattern was more rounded, harmonious, and full-bodied. She couldn't explain it yet, but she could feel it, chart it, and predict it. "Even in silence, the body speaks. And often, it speaks through sound we've been taught to ignore," she explains.

One early breakthrough came when her cousin's voice, normally energetic, began sounding flat and dull. Sharry noted the change and asked her cousin if she felt sick. Her cousin shrugged it off. Days later, she was hospitalized with appendicitis.

These moments—small, profound, and often private—shaped Sharry's belief that the voice was not merely expressive; it was diagnostic. In high school, she began to give informal talks about what she was discovering. Her peers didn't always understand her ideas, but they were intrigued. Her teachers were puzzled, unsure whether to praise her curiosity or steer her toward more traditional paths. Sharry knew she was standing at the edge of something big, even if no one else could see it yet.

This chapter of Sharry's life wasn't filled with lab coats or grants or clinical trials. It was filled with questions, cassette tapes, and intuition sharpened by relentless observation. Long before she coined terms like "Vocal Profiling" or founded an institute, Sharry was already laying the foundation for a new field—one voice at a time.

Despite resistance, Sharry pursued her questions. Lacking institutional support, she began early experiments with frequency analysis on friends and family. Her unorthodox ideas alienated traditionalists but opened the door to discoveries few had imagined.

"Sometimes, you have to build your own laboratory with nothing but questions and courage," she asserts.

During this time, Sharry enrolled in music, biology, and communications programs, hoping formal education would provide answers. But the more she studied, the more she realized her insights didn't quite fit the curriculum. Professors spoke of pitch and harmony in music theory, but not how stress affected tone. Biology classes taught about cells and organs, but not how vocal frequencies might reflect biochemical processes. So she became her own researcher, reading textbooks by day and running frequency experiments by night.

In the absence of lab equipment, she improvised. She borrowed an oscilloscope from a local repair shop and learned to use tuning forks and cassette tapes to analyze vocal fluctuations. Her kitchen table became her lab bench. Her siblings and neighbors became subjects. Patterns emerged. She discovered that people who experienced chronic fatigue often had a dip in mid-range vocal frequencies, while those with inflammation had excessive sharp spikes in the lower spectrum.

She started organizing her observations. Notebooks filled with scribbled frequency charts, symptoms, and correlations. Over time, her collection of vocal samples became a crude but valuable archive. Each tape held a story, each frequency graph was a possible roadmap to wellness.

Sharry also began attending alternative health seminars, not as a student of the systems they taught, but to test her own ideas in a broader community. She would bring recordings and charts, looking for parallels in what naturopaths and chiropractors were diagnosing manually. To her surprise, her findings often matched with their own.

Yet, gaining credibility was an uphill battle. Mainstream scientists dismissed her ideas as pseudoscience. Doctors scoffed. Grants were denied. But in her community, the people she helped spoke loudly. A woman whose chronic migraines had baffled doctors reported relief after only weeks of tone therapy. A child with severe anxiety improved dramatically when exposed to calming frequencies tuned to his vocal gaps.

"I didn't need validation," Sharry recalls. "I needed verification. And I was getting it, person by person."

It was these years of research which Sharry undertook during that time that resulted in the foundation she laid for Human BioAcoustics and the development of her proprietary computerized voice assessment approach to Vocal Profiling, all of which she achieved with a minimum of support from the medical community, the government, or private funding.

Sharry's early years were marked by determination, resilience, and a deep belief that what she was discovering mattered. She wasn't merely exploring sound—she was building a bridge between the invisible and the measurable, between voice and vitality. Her approach was grounded in one key principle:

The voice doesn't lie. It is an involuntary, real-time report of the body's state. And if it could be measured, it could be decoded. And if it could be decoded, it might be healed.

It was during a pivotal health event in her community that Sharry truly began to understand the healing potential of sound. A local man suffering from a severe neurological disorder—tremors, speech slurring, and disorientation—came to her out of desperation. After analyzing his vocal frequencies, Sharry identified patterns that suggested biochemical imbalances. She created a custom set of sound frequencies and played them back to him in short sessions. To the astonishment of everyone involved, his symptoms began to ease. This moment marked a major turning point. What had once been curiosity and personal experimentation now had measurable impact. The man's improvement wasn't subtle. It was life-changing. His muscle control returned. His speech became clearer. And Sharry, for the first time, felt the full weight of what she had been building all along: A practical method for healing based on sound.

Sharry meticulously documented the case. She recorded pre- and post-treatment voice samples, tracked the man's physical symptoms, and wrote detailed notes on the tone combinations she used for him. These weren't just casual observations; they were blueprints that led her to the realization that she needed to formalize the work she was doing. To that end, she founded her Research Institute in Albany, Ohio.

The Institute started small. Originally, it comprised just a room filled with analog equipment, computers with early spectral analysis software, and rows of cassette tapes labeled with frequencies and symptoms. But it quickly became a hub of innovation. Local residents came for help; alternative practitioners came to learn. At the Institute, Sharry began developing software that could digitize voice recordings and generate spectrograms that provided visual representations of vocal data. These voiceprints made it easier to see what she had always heard.

Over time, Sharry and her small team built a database of frequency signatures related to specific physical conditions, such as inflammation, hormonal imbalances, immune dysfunction, and nutrient deficiencies. "The voice became a roadmap. And every bump, every dip in the wave-form, was a clue the body was whispering," she recounts.

She also developed tone generators, the digital tools that produced the exact frequencies she found missing or distorted in a person's voice-print. By delivering those tones back to the client through sound therapy sessions, she could stimulate the body's natural healing processes.

Sharry also began offering training programs for those who wanted to learn her methods. Nurses, chiropractors, engineers, musicians, and holistic health practitioners came to her to learn how to decode the voice and craft frequency solutions. She called it Vocal Profiling—a term that would come to define an entirely new modality of health assessment.

Word of her work began to spread beyond the local community. Articles appeared in alternative health magazines. Practitioners shared testimonials. Sharry was invited to speak at integrative health conferences and even on public radio. While many in the traditional medical establishment remained skeptical, the results were undeniable. Eventually, what had begun as a curious girl's experiments in the foothills of Appalachia had become a pioneering force in alternative medicine. Sharry had found her frequency—not just the literal resonance that defined her work, but the deeper purpose that would shape the rest of her life.

I say without hesitation that Sharry's work represents a giant leap forward, not only in our understanding of healing, but also of our true nature as multidimensional "energy beings." The fact that energy is at the heart of all healing is not a new concept, as the healing traditions of Ayurveda and Traditional Chinese Medicine, both of which are thousands of years old, make clear. What *are* new are the exciting applications for healing energetically that Sharry is advancing using sound therapy. Thanks to her lifelong efforts and dedication to channeling her innate talents in the service of others, we now have the capability to heal ourselves in ways that goes far beyond today's common, yet all too often ineffective and, in some cases even dangerous, symptom-care approaches.

Given our nation's ever-increasing health care crisis, which now costs over $4 trillion each year, one would think that Sharry's work would be widely accepted and supported, especially by those in positions of influence who claim to be so concerned with finding viable health care solutions at a time when well over 100 Americans suffer from some form of chronic illness.

Moreover, one would hope that the work Sharry and her colleagues are doing would receive the necessary financial support that is necessary to conduct further studies, train practitioners, and make this marvelous healing technology widely available throughout our nation, and then throughout the world. All of this could be achieved with the smallest of fractions of the annual research monies given out by the National Institutes of Health (NIH) that are derived from our tax dollars.

Sadly, that is not the case.

Moreover, instead of being properly acknowledged for the work she continues to do and the breakthroughs she continues to pioneer, Sharry has been forced to labor in semi-obscurity, enduring ongoing unfair and malicious attacks that would long ago have forced most other people to give up.

But not Sharry.

No matter what, she still marshals her courage and energies and moves forward.

In my conversations with Sharry, I am always struck by two things:

Her incredible, ever-probing intelligence. And the spiritual wisdom that infuses it, keeping her humble and focused on her life-mission while so many others in the healing arts, none of whom come close to achieving breakthroughs on par with Sharry's, spend much of their time in self-promotion, dancing to the tune of their egos.

Therefore, to all of you readers who are in a position to do so, I call on you in joining me in supporting Sharry and her work. If you are writers and journalists, do what you can to spread the word about the healing breakthroughs that have been documented in this book you are reading. The American public needs to know about all that you have learned.

And to any legislators who are reading this, I urge you to stand with Sharry and the tens of millions of other Americans who advocate for medical freedom in this country, in place of the severely uneven playing field that currently exists that is dominated and controlled by those with a vested interest in keeping the status quo as it is. $4 trillion a year is a very strong compulsion for doing so, as far as they are concerned. Don't be one of their lackeys. Vote and legislate with your conscience to make sure that every American has unimpeded access, not only to Sharry's work, but to all methods of healing that go beyond the scope and understanding of our conventional medical establishment.

After all, given our nation's health statistics, it is highly likely that one day you or your loved ones may be in dire need of these breakthrough methods yourselves. So please do your part to ensure that they not only remain available to us all, but that they also receive their fair share of government funding and legislative support.

Finally, to all of the health professionals reading this, I urge you to take the training necessary to become competent in the practice of the Sound Health technologies that Sharry has developed so that you can help make them more widely available, beginning with your own clients and patients.

The age of what I call "chemical medicine" is coming to its end. Though it will always have a valid and valuable place in the healing arts, by its very nature it is unable to address healing at the causative level. That level is energy. Because of Sharry and others like her, we now know how to harness this energy to safely and effectively create medical miracles on a consistent basis. The evidence speaks for itself. Human BioAcoustics can help the body identify and reverse its own disease, often in ways that are superior to and safer than the mainstream diagnostic and therapeutic methods of conventional medicine. As such, Sharry's work is an evolutionary leap in the field of medicine and healing. And it has been my honor and privilege to assist her in writing this book.

Larry Trivieri Jr is a bestselling health book author and a recognized lay expert in the fields of self-care and holistic and integrative medicine.

www.ingramcontent.com/pod-product-compliance
Lightning Source LLC
Chambersburg PA
CBHW021902020426
42334CB00013B/440